G000024108

THE ULTIMATE ALKALINE

DIET COOKBOOK

300 RECIPES FOR YOUR HEALTH, TO LOSE WEIGHT NATURALLY AND BRING YOUR BODY BACK TO BALANCE

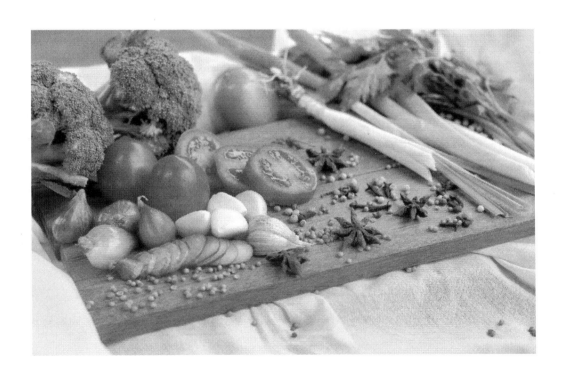

© Copyright 2020 - All rights reserved.

The content contained within this book may not be reproduced, duplicated or transmitted without direct written permission from the author or the publisher.

Under no circumstances will any blame or legal responsibility be held against the publisher, or author, for any damages, reparation, or monetary loss due to the information contained within this book. Either directly or indirectly.

Legal Notice:

This book is copyright protected. This book is only for personal use. You cannot amend, distribute, sell, use, quote or paraphrase any part, or the content within this book, without the consent of the author or publisher.

Disclaimer Notice:

Please note the information contained within this document is for educational and entertainment purposes only. All effort has been executed to present accurate, up to date, and reliable, complete information. No warranties of any kind are declared or implied. Readers acknowledge that the author is not engaging in the rendering of legal, financial, medical or professional advice. The content within this book has been derived from various sources. Please consult a licensed professional before attempting any techniques outlined in this book.

By reading this document, the reader agrees that under no circumstances is the author responsible for any losses, direct or indirect, which are incurred as a result of the use of information contained within this document, including, but not limited to, — errors, omissions, or inaccuracies.

Table of Contents

Conclusion... **206**

Introduction

The alkaline diet, or the alkaline ash diet, takes a whole new approach to what we consume. It does not consider the proportions or the nutritional composition of foods like other diets do. Instead, it considers the effects the different types of metabolic waste produce after food has been digested and assimilated. The type of food determines the nature of its metabolic waste. Therefore, food containing acid compounds or acidic elements produces acidic waste, whereas alkaline foods produce alkaline metabolic waste. The experts who first suggested the idea of an alkaline diet for healthier living say that acidic metabolic waste is harmful to bodily health as it can disrupt the optimal pH levels within the body which are essential to regulating enzyme function, hormone production, and other metabolic reactions. That is why the alkaline diet was proposed, it can help maintain the internal alkaline environment through the production of alkaline metabolic waste.

Chapter 1. About This Diet

Modern man's everyday diet has ruined our metabolic systems (along with other environmental factors), causing it to slow down and become inefficient when it comes to burning up fat from the food we eat. To help you understand that better, here's a quick summary of facts:

This "caveman" diet was based on animal foods and minimally (almost none at all) processed plants. However, as time progressed and agriculture became the main source of livelihood for man, the standard Western diet went through an immense change.

Grains aren't a typical part of our diet and our bodies, according to the Alkaline Guide, aren't meant to digest these. The same applies to milk, cheese, and other derivative products for these were only introduced after the man has learned to domesticate livestock.

Sugar and salt consumption rose towards the beginning of the Industrial revolution and in some way, our body never really got used to having too much of it-- way beyond what we can normally get from fruits and other plant food.

The diet we all have now is highly acidic and this causes numerous health problems, unsurprisingly. This is what the alkaline diet wishes to change, and wants to bring us back to what was more natural for us to consume. Resetting our metabolisms-- and making us fat-burning "machines" just like our ancestors.

Now, all of that might sound a little complicated but the further we go, the easier it will be to understand. Let's start with acidic food and how it affects our bodies.

Symptoms of a highly acidic diet include:

A lack of energy and a sensation of heaviness in your limbs. This can also include a loss of your psychic drive as well as physical tone. You might also feel depressed or an inability to cope.

You are more susceptible to different illnesses and infections.

You frequently feel cold and your body temperature has significantly lowered. You might also get frequent headaches or dizzy spells.

You have dry skin which also tends to experience irritations in areas where you sweat a lot. This is because your sweat has become highly acidic as well and if you have sensitive skin, you might feel slight burning sensations on it.

You might also experience stomach pains due to excess gastric acid or acid regurgitation. Ulcers and gastritis are also common symptoms associated with a highly acidic diet.

By switching up the food you regularly eat into something more alkaline, you would be able to avoid all of that and bring back the proper pH balance of your blood. Not to mention the fact that you'll also be helping your metabolism return to normal-- making it more efficient when it comes to burning up fat and using it for energy. That alone would hasten the process of weight loss for you.

Chapter 2. Why Is the Body Balance Important?

The primary benefit of following the alkaline diet is that it restores or at least brings the body's pH from acidic to more alkaline. Too much acidity can produce lots of health problems and an alkaline diet can help prevent these.

Other benefits of following the alkaline diet go beyond the prevention of symptoms and problems related to too much acid. The alkaline environment helps tissues to function better.

Better energy

Cells must function well for the body to produce and use energy well. Acidity interferes with proper cellular processes and reduces energy levels. By going alkaline, the cells can function better. More energy will be produced and the other cells will have more to use for their functions. This will result in higher energy levels.

Better gum and dental health

If the body is too acidic, the oral cavity is also acidic. The acidity will cause the dental enamel to erode, which will promote the formation of dental carries, plaques, and cavities. This is also among the leading causes of bad breath. The acidic environment in the mouth promotes the overgrowth of bacteria. This will cause several oral health problems such as various gum diseases. This will also increase the risk of tooth decay. Most people notice an improvement in their breath and overall dental health once they go on an alkaline diet.

Better immunity

When the various cells in the body are healthy, the immune system functions better. The integrity of the cells is great. Cellular integrity protects the cells from infections. The pathogens will find it difficult to enter and cause trouble. If the pH in the body is low (acidic), the cells will find it hard to keep their structures intact. This will allow toxins and pathogens to easily enter and cause more damage. These pathogens and toxins can easily get inside the cells and alter it. This will stimulate the development of health problems.

Cancer, for instance, starts off this way. This is also a major reason why some people more frequently get colds and other infections compared to those who follow the alkaline diet.

Reduction in inflammation and pain

Magnesium is an important mineral in the body. It also has a vital role in maintaining the body's pH balance. If the body becomes acidic, the cells will release their magnesium stores to help in neutralizing the acidity. The more acidic the body, the more magnesium is required to counter its effects. This may be ideal but magnesium does not only function for acid neutralizing. The body has so many other uses for magnesium. Using a lot for acid-neutralizing can seriously deplete the resources for the other tissues and cellular processes to use.

One of the major tissues affected is the joint. Low magnesium in the body is one of the factors that cause joint diseases and inflammatory conditions. Also, inflammation in the other tissues in the body is attributed to low magnesium stores. Eating alkaline foods that are also rich in magnesium can replenish the resources and have more for the cells to use.

It strengthens the Neurons

When neurological processes are restored and protected, you get to protect yourself from Alzheimer's Disease and memory loss. Degenerative diseases could also be prevented.

This happens because alkaline foods also contain L-Theanine, an amino acid that promotes better neurological health—and not a lot of food products can do this.

Better Weight Control

This is a culmination of all the positive effects of alkalinity in the body. The cells function better, so that energy is better distributed. Fats are used properly and the body has enough energy. This will reduce cravings and hunger cues. If the body becomes acidic, the cells will release their magnesium stores to help in neutralizing the acidity. The more acidic the body, the more magnesium is required to counter its effects. This may be ideal but magnesium does not only function for acid neutralizing. The body has so many other uses for magnesium. That means a reduction in the frequency of hunger cues and better appetite control. Fats and energy are also burned much better, reducing the risk of accumulating more fats that contribute to weight gain.

Preventing Stomach Upset

Thermogenesis, the term given to fat to energy conversion, is increased by at least 8 to 10 % when someone uses alkaline foods in his daily diet. This not only burns fat but also regulates the digestive process.

Alkaline foods also reduce intestinal gas, and could also prevent certain diseases from happening, such as ulcers, ulcerative colitis, and Chron's Disease.

Slower Aging Process

The aging process is driven by damage to cells. When cells easily degrade and repair is slow, the aging process is accelerated. If the cells can repair damage efficiently and at a faster rate, the aging process slows down. In an acidic environment, the cells get easily damaged and at a much faster rate. Repair is slowed in acidic pH. In an alkaline environment, cells do not get as much damage and when any injury gets repaired sooner.

Also, the aging process is accelerated due to oxidative stress. This is caused by the accumulation of free radicals and toxins that eat away at the cells. Acidic pH in the body supports oxidative stress. Alkaline pH helps in reducing the toxin load and oxidative stress. These promote younger-looking, healthier cells that give a younger appearance.

Perfect for Athletes

This is mainly because they know that if they eat too much fat, their bodies would suffer, and their hearts would grow weaker—and that's never a good thing because they live such active lives. Even superstars such as LeBron James have pledged allegiance to the low carb diet—so why won't you?

More so, when you adhere to these diets, it would be easy for your body to turn nutrients into ketogenic energy. If the body becomes acidic, the cells will release their magnesium stores to help in neutralizing the acidity. The more acidic the body, the more magnesium is required to counter its effects. This may be ideal but magnesium does not only function for acid neutralizing. The body has so many other uses for magnesium. When you have ketones in your system, you get to perk yourself up, and you get to have enough energy to get through the day—and help you out with whatever it is that you have to do!

Plus, when it comes to weight loss, you really cannot expect that you'd lose weight if you keep on eating too many fats and carbohydrates. It's just not right, and won't work well with what you have in mind. Since regular exercise is said to work best with the Alkaline Diets, you can keep in mind that you could make it a part of your life—so you could be sure that the diet would work.

Avoiding Chronic Inflammation

Chronic inflammation is the reason why so many diseases happen. These diseases include Type 2 Diabetes, Heart Problems, and Cancer. This so happens because grains are—you guessed it—inflammatory. While you may not see the effects right away, in time, you'd notice how your body would disintegrate, and how you'd feel like you're no longer in shape, and that your health is on the down-low. When you keep on eating grains, you're just fueling up the problem instead of working on ways to solve it.

Staying away from Auto-Immune Diseases

Take a look at it this way: Gliadin, also known as the worst kind of gluten, is responsible for affecting the pancreas, thyroids, and the entire immune system by means of releasing antibodies that aren't meant to get out yet. When these antibodies go out, auto-immune diseases come into play and one may be afflicted with diseases such as Hashimoto's Disease, type 1 diabetes, and hypothyroidism, among others.

Incidentally, research has it that Alzheimer's Disease is often triggered by high-grain diets. It releasers blockers in the brain that could break mental processes down, and therefore lead to the deterioration of the brain.

Develop a Healthy Gut

Doctors believe that the state of your gut could affect the state of your brain. After all, when you're hungry, you tend to make decisions that are not well thought out.

As you can see, your gut is in charge of a lot of things in your body—which you often fail to see in your daily life. If the body becomes acidic, the cells will release their magnesium stores to help in neutralizing the acidity. The more acidic the body, the more magnesium is required to counter its effects. This may be ideal but magnesium does not only function for acid neutralizing. The body has so many other uses for magnesium.

These things include the way you utilize fat and carbohydrates; nutrient absorption; being satiated; vitamin and neurotransmitter production; inflammation; detoxification, and immunity against diseases, amongst others.

This is also because of the vagus nerve, found in the gut, which is the longest of the 12 cranial nerves. This is the main channel between your digestive system and your nerve cells that send signals to the brain.

In short, it would be wrong for you not to take care of your gut because it would be like a way of putting your health in danger. Why? Well, because if the given processes above does not work right, you might be afflicted with certain medical conditions, such as dementia, diabetes, allergies, cancer, ADHD, asthma, and other chronic health problems.

Not only that, the clarity of your thoughts and the way you feel are also affected. When you don't eat what's right for you, you might be afflicted with anxiety, depression, or other problems that won't make life easy for you.

When your gut is healthy, your brain gets to make more serotonin—the hormone that keeps you happy and keeps your sanity in check—one that not even the best anti-depressants could give out too much, and this is why you have to make sure that you start eating right.

Avoid Vitamin-D Deficiency

Even if you consume Vitamin D, it depletes inside the body pretty fast, and acid makes depletion even faster. If the body becomes acidic, the cells will release their magnesium stores to help in neutralizing the acidity. The more acidic the body, the more magnesium is required to counter its effects. This may be ideal but magnesium does not only function for acid neutralizing. The body has so many other uses for magnesium. More so, WGA or

Wheat Germ Agglutinin also causes bacterial growth that kills Vitamin D, and damages the gut—and could do much worse to your body in the future.

Dehydration Will Be Prevented

Unlike coffee and soda, alkaline food makes an amazing drink because it keeps the body hydrated, and makes sure that dehydration is prevented. Alkaline food has moisture, which means that it has water, unlike other flavored or carbonated drinks.

You're on the Road to Feeling So Much Better

It sounds cheesy, sure, but the thing is when you adhere to these diet combination, it's like you're giving yourself the chance to feel good again.

These days, people go through a lot of things. Their lives—possibly yours, too—could turn nasty in just a second, and it would be even harder if they don't take care of their health. So, as early as now, you should consider this book a chance for you to reverse your health— for the better, of course!

Top Health Benefits from a well-balanced pH in the body

The skin has better elasticity and looks more radiant and youthful

Sleep is deeper and more restful

Abundant physical energy

Reduced frequency of suffering from colds, flu viruses, and headaches

Improved digestion

Reduced symptoms of arthritis

Reduction of overgrowth of yeast (Candida infection)

Reduced risk for osteoporosis

Improvement of mental acuity and better mental alertness

Safe, healthy, legal natural high from better hormonal and neurotransmitter levels

Chapter 3. How You Can Lose Weight Naturally?

Highly acidic foods are, in most cases, very unhealthy and can often contribute to obesity. Acid-promoting foods affect the fat-burning capabilities of your body, while also affecting that you feel hungry more often. On the other hand, alkaline-promoting foods are considered anti-inflammatory. That gives you the chance to eat the right amount of calories and feel full after eating them. All this contributes to getting your weight in order and maintaining it.

Other health benefits of a balanced alkaline diet include anti-aging effects, such as your skin being more youthful and elastic. It also increases your energy levels and your mental alertness, while securing proper digestion and better sleep at night.

First things first, it is important to understand how acidic-forming foods negatively affect our bodies; which is mainly through the red blood cells. The red blood cells have a mechanism that enables them to stay away from each other. This is basically a negative charge that keeps them separate from one another. Increased acidity in the blood can mess up this mechanism through robbing the red blood cells of the negative charge. This will lead to the red blood cells clumping up together, which will limit the levels of oxygen that enters your cells. Increased acidity in your blood; therefore, can lead to the weakening and death of red blood cells.

Now for the benefits of an alkaline diet:

Battles Fatigue

Too much acidity in your system decreases oxygen supply, which in turn decreases your cells' ability to repair and gather up nutrients. When your body lacks enough nutrients to give it energy, you will certainly feel weak. If you have been feeling tired and dazed through the day yet you had enough sleep, then you might need to check up on your acidity levels.

Boosts the immune system

An unbalance in pH lowers your body's ability to fight viruses and bacteria. Where there is lack of oxygen in the system (which acidity causes as explained above), viruses and bacteria flourish easily in the bloodstream. To eliminate the probability of diseases happening, alkalizing is essential.

Strengthens your bones

The more people age, the more the body uses up calcium especially, if you eat more acid based foods. This is because when we eat foods with high acidity, the body needs to balance the acid by dispensing calcium, magnesium and phosphorus. More than often, these minerals are taken from the bone stores, which can be a huge problem in the long run. But don't worry, with the alkaline diet, since you are not taking less of acid-forming foods, your body does not need to extract these minerals from your bones. In addition, you consume more of these minerals from the many alkaline foods high in these minerals

Healthier body and weight loss

The alkaline diet provides a base for a rather healthy diet. First, the diet requires you to cut out/reduce alcohol, red meats, sugars, trans fats and processed foods, which will definitely help you with weight loss and offer you other numerous health benefits. Also, the diet requires you to increase your intake of fresh and healthy foods such as veggies and fruits and water, which boost your general health and increase your chances of losing weight.

Chapter 4. Breakfast

Nut & Seed Granola

Preparation time: 15 minutes

Cooking time: 28 minutes.

Servings: 8

Ingredients:

- ½ cup unsweetened coconut flakes
- 1 cup raw almonds
- 1 cup raw cashews
- ¼ cup raw sunflower seeds, shelled
- ¼ cup raw pumpkin seeds, shelled
- ¼ cup coconut oil
- ½ cup maple syrup
- 1 tsp vanilla extract
- ½ cup golden raisins
- ½ cup black raisins
- Sea salt, to taste

Directions:

1. Preheat the oven to 275 F. Line a large baking sheet with parchment paper.
2. In a food processor, add the coconut flakes, almonds, cashews, and seeds and pulse until chopped finely.
3. Meanwhile, in a medium non-stick pan, add the oil, maple syrup, and vanilla extract and cook for 3 minutes over medium-high heat stirring continuously.
4. Remove from the heat and immediately stir in the nut mixture.
5. Transfer the mixture to the prepared baking sheet and spread it out evenly.
6. Bake for about 25 minutes, stirring twice.
7. Remove the pan from the oven and immediately stir in the raisins.
8. Sprinkle with a little salt.
9. With the back of a spatula, flatten the surface of the mixture.
10. Set aside to cool completely.
11. Then, break into even chunks.
12. Serve with your choice of non-dairy milk and fruit topping.
13. For preserving, transfer this granola to an airtight container and keep it in the refrigerator.

Nutrition: Calories 382; Total Fat 25 g; Saturated Fat 9.6 g; Cholesterol 0 mg; Sodium 39 mg; Total Carbs 37.9 g; Fiber 3.5 g; Sugar 24 g; Protein 7.3 g

Chia Seed Pudding

Preparation time: 10 minutes.

Servings: 2

Ingredients:

- 1 cup unsweetened almond milk
- 1/3 cup chia seeds
- 1 tsp vanilla liquid stevia
- 1 tsp organic vanilla extract
- Pinch of sea salt
- ¼ cup fresh strawberries, hulled and sliced

Directions:

1. Place all the **Ingredients:** except the strawberries in a bowl and whisk them until well combined.
2. Refrigerate the mixture for at least 10 minutes before serving.
3. Top the mixture with strawberry slices and serve.

Nutrition: Calories 218; Total Fat 13.8 g; Saturated Fat 0.2 g; Cholesterol 0 mg; Sodium 207 mg; Total Carbs 21.3 g; Fiber 16.9 g; Sugar 1.2 g; Protein 8.6 g

---

Buckwheat Porridge

Preparation time: 10 minutes.

Servings: 4

Ingredients:

- 2 cups buckwheat groats, soaked overnight and rinsed well
- 1½ cups unsweetened almond milk
- 2 tbsp chia seeds
- 1 tsp organic vanilla extract
- ¼ cup agave nectar
- 1 tsp ground cinnamon
- Pinch of sea salt
- ½ cup mixed fresh berries

Directions:

1. Place the buckwheat groats, almond milk, chia seeds and vanilla extract in a food processor and pulse until well combined.
2. Add the agave nectar, cinnamon, and salt and pulse until smooth.
3. Transfer the mixture into serving bowls and serve immediately topped with berries.
4. **Nutrition:** Calories 325; Total Fat 5.5 g; Saturated Fat 0.5 g; Cholesterol 0 mg; Sodium 133 mg; Total Carbs 65.3 g; Fiber 11.3 g; Sugar 18 g; Protein 9.6 g

Spiced Quinoa Porridge

Preparation time: 10 minutes

Cooking time: 15 minutes.

Servings: 4

Ingredients:

- 1 cup uncooked red quinoa, rinsed and drained
- 2 cups water
- ½ tsp organic vanilla extract
- ½ cup coconut milk
- ¼ tsp fresh lemon peel, grated finely
- 10-12 drops liquid stevia
- 1 tsp ground cinnamon
- ½ tsp ground ginger
- ½ tsp ground nutmeg
- Pinch of ground cloves
- ¼ cup almonds, chopped

Directions:

1. In a large pan, mix together the quinoa, water, and vanilla extract over medium heat and bring it to a boil.
2. Reduce the heat to low and simmer covered for about 15 minutes or until all the liquid is absorbed, stirring occasionally.
3. Add the coconut milk, lemon peel, stevia, and spices to the same pan and stir everything to combine.
4. Immediately, remove the pan from the heat and fluff the quinoa with a fork.
5. Divide the quinoa mixture into serving bowls evenly.
6. Top with almonds and serve.

Nutrition: Calories 265; Total Fat 12.8 g; Saturated Fat 6.9 g; Cholesterol 0 mg; Sodium 11 mg; Total Carbs 31.1 g; Fiber 4.8 g; Sugar 1.4 g; Protein 8 g

---

Fruity Oatmeal

Preparation time: 10 minutes.

Servings: 2

Ingredients:

- 1 cup rolled oats
- 1 large banana, peeled and mashed
- ¼ cup pecans, chopped
- 2 tsp chia seeds
- 1 cup unsweetened almond milk
- ¼ cup fresh blueberries
- 2 tbsp pecans, chopped

Directions:

1. Place all the **Ingredients:** except the pecans in a large bowl and mix until well combined.
2. Refrigerate, covered overnight.
3. In the morning, remove the mixture from the refrigerator and serve it topped with almonds.

Nutrition: Calories 454; Total Fat 25.1 g; Saturated Fat 2.6 g; Cholesterol 0 mg; Sodium 93 mg; Total Carbs 53 g; Fiber 11.7 g; Sugar 11.5 g; Protein 10.6 g

---

Baked Oatmeal

Preparation time: 15 minutes

Cooking time: 45 minutes. Total time: 1 hour

Servings: 6

Ingredients:

- 3 tbsp water
- 1 tbsp flax seed meal
- 3 cups unsweetened almond milk
- ¼ cup agave nectar
- 2 tbsp coconut oil, melted and cooled
- 2 tsp organic vanilla extract
- 1 tsp organic baking powder
- 1 tsp ground cinnamon
- ¼ tsp sea salt
- 2 cups old-fashioned rolled oats
- ½ cup pecans, chopped

Directions:

1. In a bowl, add the water and flax seed meal and beat until well combined.
2. Set aside.
3. Place the flax seed mixture, almond milk, agave nectar, coconut oil, vanilla extract, baking powder, cinnamon, and salt in a large bowl and beat until well combined.
4. Add the oats and pecans and stir to combine.
5. Place the oat mixture into a lightly greased 8x8-inch and spread it into an even layer.
6. Using a plastic wrap, cover the baking dish and refrigerate for no less than 8 hours or overnight.
7. Arrange a rack in the middle position of the oven and preheat the oven to 350 degrees F.
8. Remove the baking dish from the refrigerator and remove the plastic wrap.
9. With a spoon, stir the oat mixture well.
10. Bake uncovered for about 45 minutes or until the center is set.
11. Remove it from the oven and set it aside to cool slightly.
12. Serve warm with your desired toppings.

Nutrition: Calories 286; Total Fat 15.8 g; Saturated Fat 5.2 g; Cholesterol 0 mg; Sodium 17 mg; Total Carbs 32.8 g; Fiber 5.6 g; Sugar 10.9 g; Protein 5.4 g

Blueberry Pancakes

Preparation time: 10 minutes

Cooking time: 15 minutes.

Servings: 3

Ingredients:

- 1 cup rolled oats
- 1 medium banana, peeled and mashed
- ¼-½ cup unsweetened almond milk
- 1 tbsp organic baking powder
- 1 tbsp organic apple cider vinegar
- 1 tbsp agave nectar
- ½ tsp organic vanilla extract
- ½ cup fresh blueberries

Directions:

1. Place all the **Ingredients:** except the blueberries in a large bowl and mix until well combined.
2. Gently fold in the blueberries.
3. Set the mixture aside for about 5-10 minutes.
4. Preheat a large non-stick skillet over medium-low heat.
5. Add about ¼ cup of the mixture and spread in an even layer.
6. Immediately, cover the skillet and cook for about 2-3 minutes or until golden.
7. Flip the pancake over and cook for 1-2 minutes more.
8. Repeat with the remaining mixture.
9. Serve warm.

Nutrition: Calories 183; Total Fat 2.3 g; Saturated Fat 0.4 g; Cholesterol 0 mg; Sodium 22 mg; Total Carbs 38.9 g; Fiber 4.9 g; Sugar 12.6 g; Protein 4.3 g

---

Tofu & Mushroom Muffins

Preparation time: 15 minutes

Cooking time: 30 minutes.

Servings: 6

Ingredients:

- 1 tsp olive oil
- 1½ cups fresh mushrooms, chopped
- 1 scallion, chopped
- 1 tsp garlic, minced
- 1 tsp fresh rosemary, minced

- Freshly ground black pepper, to taste
- 1 (12.3 oz) package lite firm silken tofu, pressed and drained
- ¼ cup unsweetened soy milk

- 2 tbsp nutritional yeast
- 1 tbsp arrowroot starch
- 1 tsp coconut oil, softened
- ¼ tsp ground turmeric

Directions:

1. Preheat oven to 375 degrees F. Grease a 12-cup muffin pan.
2. In a non-stick skillet, heat the oil over medium heat and sauté the scallions and garlic for about 1 minute.
3. Add the mushrooms and sauté for about 5-7 minutes.
4. Stir in the rosemary and black pepper and remove from the heat.
5. Set aside to cool slightly.
6. In a food processor, add the tofu and remaining **Ingredients:** and pulse until smooth.
7. Transfer the tofu mixture to a large bowl.
8. Fold in the mushroom mixture.
9. Transfer the mixture into the prepared muffin cups evenly.
10. Bake for about 20-22 minutes or until the tops become golden brown.
11. Remove the muffin pan from the oven and place it onto a wire rack to cool for about 10 minutes.
12. Carefully, invert the muffins onto a platter and serve warm.

Nutrition: Calories 87; Total Fat 3.7 g; Saturated Fat 1.1 g; Cholesterol 0 mg; Sodium 32 mg; Total Carbs 7.4 g; Fiber 1.8 g; Sugar 2.3 g; Protein 8 g

---

Eggless Tomato "Omelet"

Preparation time: 15 minutes

Cooking time: 12 minutes.

Servings: 4

Ingredients:

- 1 cup chickpea flour
- ¼ tsp ground turmeric
- ¼ tsp red chili powder
- Pinch of ground cumin
- Pinch of sea salt
- 1½-2 cups water

- 1 medium onion, chopped finely
- 2 medium tomatoes, chopped finely
- 1 jalapeño pepper, chopped finely
- 2 tbsp fresh cilantro, chopped
- 2 tbsp olive oil, divided

Directions:

1. In a large bowl, add the flour, spices, and salt and mix well.
2. Slowly, add the water and mix until well combined.
3. Fold in the onion, tomatoes, green chili, and cilantro.
4. In a large non-stick frying pan, heat ½ tablespoon of the oil over medium heat.
5. Add ½ of the tomato mixture and tilt the pan to spread it.
6. Cook for about 5-7 minutes.
7. Place the remaining oil over the "omelet" and carefully flip it over.
8. Cook for about 4-5 minutes or until golden brown.
9. Repeat with the remaining mixture.

Nutrition: Calories 267; Total Fat 10.3 g; Saturated Fat 1.3 g; Cholesterol 0 mg; Sodium 86 mg; Total Carbs 35.7 g; Fiber 10.2 g; Sugar 8.3 g; Protein 10.6 g

---

Quinoa Bread

Preparation time: 10 minutes

Cooking time: 1½ hours. 40 minutes

Servings: 12

Ingredients:

- 1¾ cups uncooked quinoa, soaked overnight, rinsed and drained
- ¼ cup chia seeds, soaked in ½ cup of water overnight
- ½ tsp bicarbonate soda
- Sea salt, to taste
- ¼ cup olive oil
- ½ cup water
- 1 tbsp fresh lemon juice

Directions:

1. Preheat oven to 320 degrees F. Line a loaf pan with parchment paper.
2. Add all the **Ingredients:** in a food processor and pulse for about 3 minutes.
3. Place the mixture into the prepared loaf pan evenly.
4. Bake for about 1½ hours or until a toothpick inserted in the center comes out clean.
5. Remove it from the oven and place the loaf pan onto a wire rack to cool for at least 10-15 minutes.
6. Carefully, invert the bread onto the rack to cool completely before slicing.
7. With a sharp knife, cut the bread loaf into desired sized slices and serve.

Nutrition: Calories 151; Total Fat 7.2 g; Saturated Fat 0.8 g; Cholesterol 0 mg; Sodium 21 mg; Total Carbs 18.3 g; Fiber 3.8 g; Sugar 0 g; Protein 4.5 g

Raspberry Smoothie Bowl

Preparation time: 10 minutes

Servings: 2

Ingredients:

- 2 cups fresh raspberries, divided
- 2 large frozen bananas, peeled
- ½ cup unsweetened almond milk
- ⅓ cup fresh mixed berries

Directions:

1. In a blender, add the raspberries, bananas, and almond milk and pulse until smooth.
2. Transfer the smoothie into two serving bowls and top each serving with berries, serve immediately.

Nutrition: Calories 208 Total Fat 2.2 g Saturated Fat 0.3 g Cholesterol 0 mg Sodium 48 mg Total Carbs 49.1 g Fiber 2.6 g Sugar 23.7 g Protein 3.4 g

---

Chia Seed Pudding

Preparation time: 10 minutes Refrigeration time: 3 hours Total time: 3 hours and 10 minutes

Servings: 3

Ingredients:

- 2 cups unsweetened almond milk
- ½ cup chia seeds
- 1 tablespoon maple syrup
- 1 teaspoon organic vanilla extract
- ⅓ cup fresh strawberries, hulled and sliced
- 2 tablespoons almonds, sliced

Directions:

1. In a large bowl, add the almond milk, chia seeds, maple syrup, and vanilla extract and stir to combine well.
2. Refrigerate for at least 3-4 hours, stirring occasionally.
3. Serve with the strawberry and almond slice topping.

Nutrition: Calories 153 ;Total Fat 11 g; Saturated Fat 0.9 g ; Cholesterol 0 mg ; Sodium 121 mg ;Total Carbs 16.1 g ;Fiber 8.2 g; Sugar 5.1 g; Protein 5.6 g

Spiced Quinoa Porridge

Preparation time: 10 minutes

Cooking time: 15 minutes

Servings: 4

Ingredients:

- 1 cup uncooked red quinoa, rinsed and drained
- 2 cups water
- ½ teaspoon organic vanilla extract
- ½ cup coconut milk
- ¼ teaspoon fresh lemon peel, grated finely
- 10-12 drops liquid stevia
- 1 teaspoon ground cinnamon
- ½ teaspoon ground ginger
- ½ teaspoon ground nutmeg
- Pinch of ground cloves
- 2 tablespoons almonds, chopped

Directions:

1. In a large pan, mix together the quinoa, water, and vanilla extract over medium heat and bring to a boil.
2. Reduce the heat to low and simmer, covered for about 15 minutes or until all the liquid is absorbed, stirring occasionally.
3. In the pan with the quinoa, add the coconut milk, lemon peel, stevia, and spices and stir to combine.
4. Immediately remove from the heat and fluff the quinoa with a fork.
5. Divide the quinoa mixture evenly into serving bowls.
6. Serve with a topping of chopped almonds.

Nutrition: Calories 248 Total Fat 11.4 g Saturated Fat 6.8 g Cholesterol 0 mg Sodium 11 mg Total Carbs 30.5 g Fiber 4.4 g Sugar 1.3 g Protein 7.4 g

---

Buckwheat Porridge

Preparation time: 15 minutes

Cooking time: 7 minutes

Servings: 2

Ingredients:

- ½ cup buckwheat groats
- 2 tablespoons chia seeds
- 15-20 almonds
- 1 cup unsweetened almond milk
- ½ teaspoon ground cinnamon
- 1 teaspoon organic vanilla extract
- 3-4 drops liquid stevia
- ¼ cup mixed fresh berries

Directions:

1. In a large bowl, soak buckwheat groats in 1 cup of water overnight.
2. In another 2 bowls, soak chia seeds and almonds respectively.
3. Drain the buckwheat and rinse well.
4. In a non-stick pan, add the buckwheat and almond milk over medium heat and cook for about 7 minutes or until creamy.
5. Drain the chia sees and almonds well.
6. Remove the pan from heat and stir in the almonds, chia seeds, cinnamon, vanilla extract, and stevia.
7. Serve hot with a topping of berries.

Nutrition:

Calories 282 ;Total Fat 11.4 g ;Saturated Fat 1 g ;Cholesterol 0 mg ;Sodium 97 mg ;Total Carbs 41.5 g ;Fiber 8.6 g ;Sugar 11.8 g ;Protein 8.8 g

---

Overnight Fruity Oatmeal

Preparation time: 10 minutes Refrigeration time: 12 hours Total time: 12 hours 10 minutes

Servings: 2

Ingredients:

- 1 cup rolled oats
- 1 large banana, peeled and mashed
- 3 teaspoons chia seeds
- 1 cup unsweetened almond milk
- ¼ cup fresh blueberries
- 2 tablespoons walnuts, chopped

Directions:

1. In a large bowl, add all the **Ingredients:** except for sliced blueberries and walnuts and mix well until combined.
2. Cover the bowl and refrigerate overnight.
3. Top with blueberries and walnuts and serve.

Nutrition: Calories 309 Total Fat 10.6 g Saturated Fat 1 g Cholesterol 0 mg Sodium 93 mg Total Carbs 49.1 g Fiber 8.6 g Sugar 10.6 g Protein 9.4 g

Banana Waffles

Preparation time: 15 minutes

Cooking time: 20 minutes

Servings: 5

Ingredients:

- 2 tablespoons flax meal
- 6 tablespoons warm water
- 2 bananas, peeled and mashed
- 1 cup creamy almond butter
- ¼ cup full-fat coconut milk

Directions:

1. In a small bowl, add the flax meal and warm water and beat until well combined.
2. Set aside for about 10 minutes or until mixture becomes thick.
3. In a medium mixing bowl, add the bananas, almond butter, and coconut milk, mix well.
4. Add the flax meal mixture and mix until well combined.
5. Preheat the waffle iron and lightly grease it.
6. Place desired amount of the mixture in the preheated waffle iron.
7. Cook for about 3-4 minutes or until waffles become golden brown.
8. Repeat with the remaining mixture.
9. Serve warm.

Nutrition: Calories 350 Total Fat 29.2 g Saturated Fat 3.2 g Cholesterol 0 mg Sodium 179 mg Total Carbs 21.6 g Fiber 8.4 g Sugar 9.2 g Protein 12.5 g

---

Buckwheat Pancakes

Preparation time: 15 minutes

Cooking time: 15 minutes

Servings: 5

Ingredients:

- 1 cup coconut milk
- 2 teaspoons apple cider vinegar
- 1 cup buckwheat flour
- 2 tablespoons ground flax seed
- 1 tablespoon baking powder
- ¼ teaspoon sea salt
- ¼ cup maple syrup
- 1 teaspoon vanilla extract
- 1 tablespoon coconut oil

Directions:

1. In a medium bowl, mix together the coconut milk and vinegar. Set aside.
2. In a large bowl, mix together the flour, flax seed, baking powder, and salt.
3. Add the coconut milk mixture, maple syrup, and vanilla extract and beat until well combined.
4. In a large non-stick skillet, melt the coconut oil over medium heat.
5. Place about ⅓ cup of the mixture and spread in an even circle.
6. Cook for about 1-2 minutes.
7. Flip and cook for an additional 1 minute then remove from pan.
8. Repeat with the remaining mixture.
9. Serve warm.

Nutrition: Calories 276 Total Fat 15.8 g Saturated Fat 12.8 g Cholesterol 0 mg Sodium 109 mg Total Carbs 32.5 g Fiber 4.3 g Sugar 11.8 g Protein 4.7 g

---

Tomato Omelette

Preparation time: 15 minutes

Cooking time: 25 minutes

Servings: 4

Ingredients:

- 1 cup chickpea flour
- ¼ teaspoon ground turmeric
- ¼ teaspoon red chili powder
- Pinch of ground cumin
- Pinch of salt
- 1½-2 cups water
- 1 medium onion, chopped finely
- 2 medium tomatoes, chopped finely
- 1 jalapeño pepper, chopped finely
- 2 tablespoons fresh cilantro, chopped
- 2 tablespoons olive oil, divided

Directions:

1. In a large bowl, mix together the flour, spices, and salt.
2. Slowly add the water and mix until well combined.
3. Add the onion, tomatoes, green chili, and cilantro and gently stir to combine.
4. In a large non-stick frying pan, heat ½ tablespoon of oil over medium heat.
5. Add ½ of tomato mixture and tilt the pan to spread it.
6. Cook for 5-7 minutes.
7. Pour remaining oil over the omelette and carefully flip to the other side.

8. Cook for 4-5 minutes or until golden brown and remove from pan.
9. Repeat with remaining mixture.

Nutrition: Calories 267 Total Fat 10.3 g Saturated Fat 1.3 g Cholesterol 0 mg Sodium 57 mg Total Carbs 35.7 g Fiber 10.7 g Sugar 8.3 g Protein 10.7 g

---

Tofu & Mushroom Muffins

Preparation time: 15 minutes

Cooking time: 30 minutes

Servings: 6

Ingredients:

- 1 teaspoon olive oil
- 1½ cups fresh mushrooms, chopped
- 1 scallion, chopped
- 1 teaspoon garlic, minced
- 1 teaspoon fresh rosemary, minced
- Freshly ground black pepper, to taste
- 1 (12.3-ounce) package firm silken tofu, drained
- ¼ cup unsweetened almond milk
- 2 tablespoons nutritional yeast
- 1 tablespoon arrowroot starch
- ¼ teaspoon ground turmeric
- 1 teaspoon coconut oil, softened

Directions:

1. Preheat the oven to 375 degrees F. Grease a 12-cup muffin pan.
2. In a non-stick skillet, heat oil over medium heat and sauté scallion and garlic for about 1 minute.
3. Add the mushrooms and sauté for 5-7 minutes.
4. Stir in the rosemary and black pepper and remove from the heat.
5. Set aside to cool slightly.
6. In a food processor, add the tofu and remaining **Ingredients:** and pulse until smooth.
7. Transfer the tofu mixture into a large bowl.
8. Fold in the mushroom mixture.
9. Pour the batter into prepared muffin cups evenly.
10. Bake for 20-22 minutes or until a toothpick inserted in the center comes out clean.
11. Remove the muffin pan from the oven and place onto a wire rack to cool for about 10 minutes.
12. Carefully invert the muffins onto the wire rack and serve warm.

Nutrition: Calories 84 Total Fat 3.7 g Saturated Fat 1.1 g Cholesterol 0 mg Sodium 35 mg Total Carbs 6.8 g Fiber 1.8 g Sugar 1.9 g Protein 7.7 g

Quinoa Bread 2

Preparation time: 10 minutes

Cooking time: 1 hour 30 minutes 40 minutes

Servings: 12

Ingredients:

- 1¾ cups uncooked quinoa, soaked overnight and rinsed
- ¼ cup chia seeds, soaked in ½ cup of water overnight
- ½ teaspoon bicarbonate soda
- ¼ teaspoon sea salt
- ¼ cup olive oil
- ½ cup water
- 1 tablespoon fresh lemon juice

Directions:

1. Preheat the oven to 320 degrees F. Line a loaf pan with parchment paper.
2. In a food processor, add all the **Ingredients:** and pulse for about 3 minutes.
3. Pour the mixture into prepared loaf pan evenly.
4. Bake for 1½ hours.
5. Remove the bread pan from the oven and place onto a wire rack to cool for about 10 minutes.
6. Now, invert the bread onto the wire rack to cool fully before slicing.
7. With a sharp knife, slice each bread loaf to the desired sized slices and serve.

Nutrition: Calories 137 Total Fat 6.5 g Saturated Fat 0.9 g Cholesterol 0 mg Sodium 48 mg Total Carbs 16.9 g Fiber 2.6 g Sugar 0 g Protein 4 g

---

Baked Oatmeal

Preparation time: 15 minutes

Cooking time: 45 minutes

Servings: 5

Ingredients:

- 1 tablespoon flaxseed meal
- 3 tablespoons water
- 3 cups unsweetened almond milk
- ¼ cup maple syrup
- 2 tablespoons coconut oil, melted and cooled
- 2 teaspoons organic vanilla extract
- 1 teaspoon ground cinnamon
- 1 teaspoon organic baking powder
- ¼ teaspoon salt
- 2 cups old-fashioned rolled oats

- 1 cup mixed nuts, chopped

Directions:
1. Lightly grease an 8x8-inch baking dish. Set aside.
2. In a large bowl, add the flaxseed meal and water and beat until well combined. Set aside for about 5 minutes.
3. In the bowl of flax mixture, add the remaining **Ingredients:** except the oats and nuts and mix until well combined.
4. Add the oats and nuts and gently stir to combine.
5. Place the mixture into the prepared baking dish and spread in an even layer.
6. Cover the baking dish with plastic wrap and refrigerate for about 8 hours.
7. Preheat the oven to 350 degrees F. Arrange a rack in the middle of the oven.
8. Remove the baking dish from the refrigerator and let sit at room temperature for 15-20 minutes.
9. Remove the plastic wrap and stir the oatmeal mixture well.
10. Bake for 45 minutes.
11. Remove from the oven and serve warm.

Nutrition: Calories 423 Total Fat 26.3 g Saturated Fat 7.9 g Cholesterol 0 mg Sodium 317 mg Total Carbs 41.2 g Fiber 6 g Sugar 11.2 g Protein 9.6 g

<u>Coconut & Nut Granola</u>

Preparation time: 10 minutes

Cooking time: 20 minutes

Servings: 12

Ingredients:

- 3 cups unsweetened coconut flakes
- 1 cup walnuts, chopped
- ½ cup flaxseeds
- ⅔ cup pumpkin seeds
- ⅔ cup sunflower seeds
- ¼ cup coconut oil, melted
- 1 teaspoon ground ginger
- 1 teaspoon ground cinnamon
- ⅛ teaspoon ground cloves
- ⅛ teaspoon ground cardamom
- Pinch of salt

Directions:

1. Preheat the oven to 350 degrees F. Lightly grease a large, rimmed baking sheet.
2. In a bowl, add the coconut flakes, walnuts, flaxseeds, pumpkin seeds, sunflower seeds, coconut oil, spices, and salt and toss to coat well.
3. Transfer the mixture onto the prepared baking sheet and spread in an even layer.
4. Bake for about 20 minutes, stirring after every 3-4 minutes.

5. Remove the baking sheet from the oven and let the granola cool completely before serving.
6. Break the granola into desired sized chunks and serve with your favorite non-dairy milk.

Nutrition: Calories 256 Total Fat 23 g Saturated Fat 10.3 g Cholesterol 0 mg Sodium 15 mg Total Carbs 8.5 g Fiber 4.6 g Sugar 0.3 g Protein 4.8 g

---

Crunchy Quinoa Meal

Preparation time: 5 minutes

Cooking time: 25 minutes

Servings: 2

Ingredients:

- 3 cups almond milk
- 1 cup quinoa, rinsed
- 1/8 teaspoon ground cinnamon
- 1 cup raspberry
- ½ cup chopped almonds

Directions:

1. Add milk into a saucepan and bring to a boil over high heat.
2. Add quinoa to the milk and again bring it to a boil.
3. Let it simmer for 15 minutes, on low heat until milk is reduced.
4. Stir in cinnamon and mix well.
5. Cover and cook for 8 minutes until milk is completely absorbed.
6. Add raspberry and cook for 30 seconds.
7. Serve and enjoy.

Nutrition: Calories 271 Total Fat 3.7 g Saturated Fat 2.7 g Cholesterol 168 mg Sodium 121 mg Total Carbs 54 g Fiber 3.5 g Sugar 2.3 g Protein 6.5 g

---

Almond Pancakes

Preparation time: 5 minutes

Cooking time: 15 minutes

Servings: 4

Ingredients:

- 1 cup almond flour
- 2 tablespoons arrowroot powder

- 1 teaspoon baking powder
- 1 cup almond milk
- 3 tablespoons coconut oil

Directions:

1. Mix all dry **Ingredients:** in a medium container.
2. Add almond milk and 2 tablespoons coconut oil. Mix well.
3. Melt a teaspoon coconut oil in a skillet.
4. Pour a ladle of the batter into the skillet and swirl the pan to spread it into a smooth pancake.
5. Cook for 3 minutes on low heat until firm.
6. Flip the pancake and cook for another 2 to 3 minutes until golden brown.
7. Cook more pancakes using the remaining batter.
8. Serve.

Nutrition: Calories 377 Total Fat 14.9 g Saturated Fat 4.7 g Cholesterol 194 mg Sodium 607 mg Total Carbs 60.7 g Fiber 1.4 g Sugar 3.3 g Protein 6.4g

---

Quinoa Porridge

Preparation time: 5 minutes

Cooking time: 25 minutes

Servings: 2

Ingredients:

- 2 cups almond milk
- 1 cup quinoa, rinsed
- 1/8 teaspoon ground cinnamon
- 1 cup (1/2 pint) fresh blueberries

Directions:

1. Boil almond milk in a saucepan over high heat.
2. Add quinoa to the milk and again bring it to a boil.
3. Let it simmer for 15 minutes on low heat until milk is reduced.
4. Stir in cinnamon and mix well.
5. Cover and cook for 8 mins until milk is completely absorbed.
6. Add blueberries and cook for 30 seconds.
7. Serve and enjoy.

Nutrition: Calories 271 Total Fat 3.7 g Saturated Fat 2.7 g Cholesterol 168 mg Sodium 121 mg Total Carbs 54 g Fiber 3.5 g Sugar 2.3 g Protein 6.5

Amaranth Porridge

Preparation time: 05 minutes

Cooking time: 30 minutes

Servings: 2

Ingredients:

- 2 cups almond milk
- 2 cups alkaline water
- 1 cup amaranth
- 2 tablespoons coconut oil
- 1 tablespoon ground cinnamon

Directions:

1. Mix milk with water in a medium saucepan.
2. Bring the mixture to a boil.
3. Stir in amaranth then reduce the heat to low.
4. Cook on low simmer for 30 minutes with occasional stirring.
5. Turn off the heat. Stir in cinnamon and coconut oil.
6. Serve warm.

Nutrition:

Calories 434 Total Fat 35 g Saturated Fat 0 g Cholesterol 0 mg Sodium 3 mg Total Carbs 27 gFiber 3.6 g Sugar 5.5 Protein 6.7

Banana Barley Porridge

Preparation time: 15 minutes

Cooking time: 5 minutes

Servings: 2

Ingredients:

- 1 cup unsweetened almond milk, divided
- 1 small banana, peeled and sliced
- ½ cup barley
- 3 drops liquid stevia
- ¼ cup almonds, chopped

Directions:

1. Mix barley with half almond milk and stevia in a bowl and mix well.
2. Cover and refrigerate for about 6 hours.
3. Mix the barley mixture with almond milk in a saucepan.
4. Cook for 5 minutes on medium heat.

5. Top with chopped almonds and banana slices.
6. Serve.

Nutrition: Calories 159 Total Fat 8.4 g Saturated Fat 0.7 g Cholesterol 0 mg Total Carbs 19.8 g Dietary Fiber 4.1 g Sugar 6.7 g Protein 4.6 g

---

Zucchini Muffins

Preparation time: 10 minutes

Cooking time: 25 minutes

Servings: 16

Ingredients:

- 1 tablespoon ground flaxseed
- 3 tablespoons alkaline water
- ¼ cup almond butter
- 3 small-medium over-ripe bananas
- 2 small zucchinis, grated
- ½ cup almond milk
- 1 teaspoon vanilla extract
- 2 cups almond flour
- 1 tablespoon baking powder
- 1 teaspoon cinnamon
- ¼ teaspoon sea salt
- Optional addins:
- ¼ cup chocolate chips and/or walnuts

Directions:

1. Set your oven to 375 degrees F. Grease a muffin tray with cooking spray.
2. Mix flaxseed with water in a bowl.
3. Mash bananas in a glass bowl and stir in all the remaining **Ingredients:**.
4. Mix well and divide the mixture into the muffin tray.
5. Bake for 25 minutes.
6. Serve.

Nutrition: Calories 127 Total Fat 6.6 g Saturated Fat 1.1 g Cholesterol 0 mg Sodium 292 mg Total Carbs 13 g Fiber 0.7 g Sugar 1.2 g Protein 3.8 g

Millet Porridge

Preparation time: 10 minutes

Cooking time: 20 minutes

Servings: 2

Ingredients:

- Pinch of sea salt
- 1 tablespoon almonds, chopped finely
- ½ cup unsweetened almond milk
- ½ cup millet, rinsed and drained
- 1½ cups alkaline water
- 3 drops liquid stevia

Directions:

1. Sauté millet in a non-stick skillet for 3 minutes.
2. Stir in salt and water. Let it boil then reduce the heat.
3. Cook for 15 minutes then stirs in remaining **Ingredients:**.
4. Cook for another 4 minutes.
5. Serve with chopped nuts on top.

Nutrition:

Calories 219 Total Fat 4.5 g Saturated Fat 0.6 g Cholesterol 0 mg Total Carbs 38.2 g Fiber 5 g Sugar 0.6 g Protein 6.4 g

---

Tofu Vegetable Fry

Preparation time: 10 minutes

Cooking time: 15 minutes

Servings: 4

Ingredients:

- 2 small onions, finely chopped-chopped
- 2 cups cherry tomatoes, finely chopped-chopped
- 1/8 teaspoon ground turmeric
- 1 tablespoon olive oil
- 2 red bell peppers, seeded and chopped-chopped
- 3 cups firm tofu, crumbled and chopped-chopped
- 1/8 teaspoon cayenne pepper
- 2 tablespoons fresh basil leaves, chopped-chopped
- Salt, to taste

Directions:

1. Sauté onions and bell peppers in a greased skillet for 5 minutes.
2. Stir in tomatoes and cook for 2 minutes.
3. Add turmeric, salt, cayenne pepper, and tofu.
4. Cook for 8 minutes.
5. Garnish with basil leaves.
6. Serve warm.

Nutrition:

Calories 212 Total Fat 11.8 g Saturated Fat 2.2 g Cholesterol 0 mg Total Carbs 14.6 g Dietary Fiber 4.4 g Sugar 8 g Protein 17.3 g

---

Zucchini Pancakes

Preparation time: 15 minutes

Cooking time: 8 minutes

Servings: 8

Ingredients:

- 12 tablespoons alkaline water
- 6 large zucchinis, grated
- Sea salt, to taste
- 4 tablespoons ground Flax Seeds
- 2 teaspoons olive oil
- 2 jalapeño peppers, finely chopped
- ½ cup scallions, finely chopped

Directions:

1. Mix together water and flax seeds in a bowl and keep aside.
2. Heat oil in a large non-stick skillet on medium heat and add zucchini, salt, and black pepper.
3. Cook for about 3 minutes and transfer the zucchini into a large bowl.
4. Stir in scallions and flax seed mixture and thoroughly mix.
5. Preheat a griddle and grease it lightly with cooking spray.
6. Pour about ¼ of the zucchini mixture into preheated griddle and cook for about 3 minutes.
7. Flip the side carefully and cook for about 2 more minutes.
8. Repeat with the remaining mixture in batches and serve.

Nutrition: Calories 71 Total Fat 2.8 g Saturated Fat 0.4 g Cholesterol 0 mg Total Carbs 9.8 g Dietary Fiber 3.9 g Sugar 4.5 g Protein 3.7 g

Pumpkin Spice Quinoa

Preparation time: 10 minutes

Cooking time: 0minutes

Servings: 02

Ingredients:

- 1 cup cooked quinoa
- 1 cup unsweetened almond milk
- 1 large banana, mashed
- 1/4 cup pumpkin puree
- 1 teaspoon pumpkin spice
- 2 teaspoon chia seeds

Directions:

1. Mix all the **Ingredients:** in a container.
2. Seal the lid and shake well to mix.
3. Refrigerate overnight.
4. Serve.

Nutrition: Calories 212 Total Fat 11.9 g Saturated Fat 02 g Cholesterol 112 mg Sodium 125 mg Total Carbs 31.7 g Fiber 2 g Sugar 2.3 g Protein 7.3g

---

Chia Parfait

Ingredients:

- Diced mango (.25 c.)
- Mashed raspberries (.25 c.)
- Coconut flakes (1 Tbsp.)
- Chopped cashews (2 Tbsp.)
- Nutmeg (.25 tsp.)
- Cinnamon (.25 tsp.)
- Vanilla (.5 tsp.)
- Chia seeds (3 Tbsp.)
- Almond milk (.75 c.)

Directions:

1. To start this recipe, take the cashews, nutmeg, cinnamon, vanilla, chia seeds, and almond milk.
2. Let this sit overnight in the glass jar in the fridge overnight.
3. In the morning, layer on the coconut flakes, mango, and raspberries and then serve.

Warm Apple Pie Cereal

Ingredients:

- Maple syrup (1 tsp.)
- Chopped raw almonds (.25 c.)
- Diced Granny Smith apple (1)
- Raisins (.25 c.)
- Juiced lemon (.5)
- Pinch of nutmeg
- Pinch of allspice
- Cinnamon (.5 tsp.)
- Vanilla (.25 tsp.)
- Almond milk, unsweetened (1.5 c.)
- Quinoa (.5 c.)

Directions:

1. To start, take the quinoa, almond milk, vanilla, cinnamon, allspice, nutmeg, juiced lemon, raisins, and apple into a pan and turn it on to medium heat.
2. Bring this to a gentle simmer and then reduce the heat to low. Cook until the quinoa is fluffy and the liquid is all gone.
3. Move this over to the serving bowl you want to use and then top with the maple syrup and almonds.

Tofu Scramble

Ingredients:

- Sliced avocado (1)
- Cilantro (1 Tbsp.)
- Water (3 Tbsp.)
- Pepper
- Salt
- Nutritional yeast (.5 c.)
- Turmeric (.5 tsp.)
- Cumin (.5 tsp.)
- Cubed tofu, firm (.5 block)
- Broccoli (1 c.)
- Sliced shallots (2)
- Red bell pepper (1)
- Olive oil (1 Tbsp.)

Directions:

1. To start this recipe, take some oil and add it to a skillet. Let it heat up before adding in the bell pepper, shallots, and broccoli.
2. After a few minutes of cooking this, add the tofu into this mixture, crumbling it up with a spoon. Cook for a bit longer.
3. While those **Ingredients:** are cooking, mix together the water, yeast, turmeric, pepper, cumin, salt, paprika and toss around to coat.
4. Add this to a skillet and coat well. Cook this all until you are out of liquid and then add the cilantro.

5. Move this all over to a plate, making sure to top with the prepared avocado and serve.

Sweet Potato Parfait

Ingredients:

- Coconut flakes (1 Tbsp.)
- Chopped walnuts (1 Tbsp.)
- Sweet potato, remove the flesh (1)
- Cinnamon .25 tsp.)
- Nutmeg (.25 tsp.)
- Grated ginger (.5 tsp.)
- Raw honey (1 tsp.)
- Plain yogurt (1 c.)

Directions:

1. When you are ready to start, take .75 cup of the yogurt and mix it with the nutmeg, ginger, and cinnamon. Set this to the side.
2. While the cooked sweet potato is warm, mash up the potato a bit.
3. In a bowl or a jar, add in the potato on the bottom. Add in some yogurt, a few walnuts, and coconut flakes.
4. Repeat these layers until you have used up all of the **Ingredients:**.

Tofu Morning Sandwich

Ingredients:

- Sliced avocado (1)
- Toasted sprouted bread (2 slices)
- Nutritional yeast (3 Tbsp.)
- Water (2 Tbsp.)
- Pepper
- Salt
- Garlic powder (1 tsp.)
- Dried oregano (1 tsp.)
- Turmeric (1 tsp.)
- Tofu (.5 block)
- Sliced shallot (1)
- Chopped broccoli (.5 c.)
- Coconut oil (1 tsp.)

Directions:

1. Bring out a big skillet and heat up your oil inside. When the oil is nice and warm, add in the shallot and broccoli. Crumble in the tofu and let it warm up.
2. While that is cooking, take out a bowl and combine together half the yeast with the water, pepper, salt, garlic, oregano, and turmeric.
3. Add this spice mixture into the broccoli and tofu mixture and then cook until the liquid has time to absorb.

4. Spoon this mixture on top of the toasted bread along with the avocado and the rest of the nutritional yeast.

Nutty Overnight Oats

Ingredients:

- Hemp hearts (1 Tbsp)
- Chopped Granny Smith apple (1)
- Almond butter (2 Tbsp.)
- Salt (.25 tsp.)
- Nutmeg (1 tsp.)
- Cinnamon (1 tsp.)
- Vanilla (1 tsp.)
- Unsweetened almond milk (2 c.)
- Uncooked oats (1 c.)

Directions:

1. Take out a bowl and combine together the salt, nutmeg, cinnamon, vanilla, almond milk, and oats.
2. When this mixture is done, divide it up into two jars and shake around a bit. Place into the fridge overnight.
3. When it is time to eat this oatmeal, add in the hemp hearts, chopped apple, and almond butter to the jars before serving.

Sunnyside Breakfast Bowl

Ingredients:

- Toasted pumpkin seeds (2 Tbsp.)
- Breakfast radish (1 sliced)
- Sliced avocado (1)
- Sliced scallions (2)
- Halved grape tomatoes (.5 c.)
- Salt (.5 tsp.)
- Water (3 c.)
- Yellow split peas (.75 c.)
- Sliced kale, bunch (.5)
- Minced garlic cloves (2)
- Diced shallots (2)
- Turmeric 1 tsp.)
- Coconut oil (1 Tbsp.)

Directions:

1. Take out a pan and place the coconut oil inside to heat up. When the oil is warm, you can add in the kale, garlic, shallots, and turmeric.
2. Cook these until the kale has time to wilt and then add in the split peas to cook for a bit.
3. Pour the salt and water into the pan and then bring it to a boil. Reduce the heat a bit and then let this all simmer together for a bit.

4. After ten minutes, you can divide up the mixture between a few bowls. Top this with some pumpkin seeds, radish, avocado, scallions, and tomatoes before serving.

Breakfast Fruit Crepes

Ingredients:

- Cacao nibs (1 Tbsp.)
- Raspberries (2 c.)
- Cashew butter (.33 c.)
- Melted ghee (2 Tbsp.)
- Water (2 c.)
- Cinnamon (.25 tsp.)
- Vanilla (.5 tsp.)
- Coconut sugar (.5 tsp.)
- Salt (.5 tsp.)
- Melted coconut oil (1 Tbsp.)
- Buckwheat flour (1 c.)
- Water (6 Tbsp.)
- Ground flax (2 Tbsp.)

Directions:

1. Take out a bowl and whisk together the water and the ground flax. Place this into the fridge to set for a bit until you see a gel form.
2. After this is done, place this mixture into the blender along with the cinnamon, vanilla, sugar, salt, coconut oil, buckwheat, and two cups of water.
3. Blend the mixture well and then set aside.
4. Add the ghee to a skillet and place on medium-low heat. Add in some of the batters to the pan, swirling it around to make a layer that is even.
5. Let this cook for a few minutes until done. And then remove from the skillet before repeating these steps. Finish up all of the batters.
6. When the crepes have a moment to cool, add in some of the cacao nibs, raspberries, and cashew butter before serving.

Fruity Breakfast Salad

Ingredients:

- Raw honey (1 tsp.)
- Lime zest (1 Tbsp.)
- Unsweetened yogurt (.5 c.)
- Crushed almonds (1 Tbsp.)
- Pomegranate seeds (.25 c.)
- Sliced blood orange (1)
- Sliced persimmon fruit (1)

Directions:

1. To start this recipe, bring out a bowl and combine together the almonds, pomegranate seeds, blood orange, and persimmon.

2. Divide this mixture between two plates evenly.
3. Take out a smaller bowl and whisk together the honey, lime zest, and yogurt.
4. Top each plate with some of the yogurt mixtures before serving.

Mocha Pudding

Ingredients:

- Raw cacao nibs (1 Tbsp.)
- Raspberries (.25 c.)
- Sliced banana (.5)
- Cinnamon (1 tsp.)
- Raw cacao (1 tsp)
- Brewed coffee (2 Tbsp.)
- Chia seeds (.25 c.)
- Vanilla (.5 tsp.)
- Almond milk (1 c.)

Directions:

1. To start this recipe, bring out a bowl and combine the cinnamon, cacao, coffee, chia seeds, vanilla, and almond milk.
2. Stir this together in order to combine, add a lid to the bowl, and place in the fridge overnight.
3. The next day, when you are ready to eat this dish, top it with the cacao nibs, raspberries, and banana and then serve.

Broccoli Omelet

Ingredients:

- Green onions (2 Tbsp.)
- Crushed pepper (.25 tsp.)
- Turmeric (.25 tsp.)
- Dijon mustard (1 tsp.)
- Tapioca starch (3 Tbsp.)
- Nutritional yeast (3 Tbsp.)
- Unsweetened almond milk (3 Tbsp.)
- Tofu, firm (12 oz.)
- The filling
- Nutritional yeast (2 Tbsp.)
- Sliced shallot (1)
- Steamed broccoli (1 c.)

Directions:

1. To start this recipe, bring out a blender and mix together the pepper, turmeric, mustard, tapioca, nutritional yeast, almond milk, and tofu.
2. Heat up a skillet until it is really hot, and then pour this batter into the skillet to cook.

3. After 7 minutes, this part will be done. Place the **Ingredients:** for the filling on one side of the omelet and then flip it over to the other side to cover.
4. Cook a bit longer before moving to a plate and garnishing with green onions to enjoy.

Tofu and Kale Tacos

Ingredients:

- Sliced avocado (1)
- Chopped cilantro (1 Tbsp.)
- Greed onions, sliced (1 Tbsp.)
- Warmed corn tortillas (4)
- Halved cherry tomatoes (5)
- Sliced kale (1 c.)
- Coconut aminos (1 Tbsp.)
- Turmeric (.25 tsp.)
- Onion powder (1 tsp.)
- Nutritional yeast (2 Tbsp.)
- Tofu (7 oz.)
- Coconut oil (1 Tbsp.)

How to use:

1. To start this recipe, bring out a skillet and heat up the coconut oil inside. When the oil is warm, add in the coconut aminos, turmeric, onion powder, and nutritional yeast with the tofu.
2. After cooking for 5 minutes, you can add in the cherry tomatoes and the kale and cook for a bit longer.
3. Take this kale and tofu mixture off the stove and divide up among the four corn tortillas.
4. Top this with the avocado, cilantro, and green onions before serving.

Savory Breakfast Bowl

Ingredients:

- Sliced green onion (1 Tbsp.)
- Cooked lentils (.33 c.)
- Red chili flakes (.25 tsp.)
- Turmeric (.5 tsp.)
- Lemon zest (1 tsp.)
- Nutritional yeast (1 Tbsp.)
- Spinach (1 c.)
- Pepper (.25 tsp.)
- Salt (.25 tsp.)
- Water (.5 c.)
- Unsweetened almond milk (.5 c.)
- Rolled oats (.5 c.)

Directions:

1. Take out a pan and heat up the pepper, salt, water, almond milk, and oats inside.

2. Let these reach a boil before reducing the heat to a simmer to cook for a bit. After five to ten minutes, the liquid should be mostly absorbed.
3. When this happens, stir in the lentils, chili flakes, turmeric, lemon zest, nutritional yeast, and spinach.
4. Take off the stove and then garnish with some green onions before you serve.

Almond Butter and Jelly Overnight Oats

Ingredients:

- Sliced raspberries (4)
- Sliced almonds (1 Tbsp.)
- Almond butter (1 Tbsp.)
- Chia seeds (1 tsp.)
- Vanilla (.5 tsp.)
- Almond milk (.75 c.)
- Rolled oats (.5 c.)
- For the jam
- Chia seeds (1 Tbsp.)
- Honey (1 tsp.)
- Mashed raspberries (.25 c.)

Directions:

1. To start this recipe, take .25 cup of mashed raspberries and combine with the tablespoon of the chia seeds with the honey.
2. Combine these Ingredients: together well and then put into the fridge to set for a bit.
3. After ten minutes, add in a tablespoon of this raspberry mixture with the chia seeds, vanilla, almond milk, and oats into a jar. Mix the Ingredients: together well.
4. Cover the jar and let it set in the fridge for 8 hours or more.
5. When it is time to serve the next day, add in the almond butter, the rest of the raspberries, and the almonds before serving.

Blueberry Muffins

Servings: 8 muffins

Ingredients:

- 1 cup hemp milk
- 3/4 cup teff flour
- 1/3 cup agave
- 1/2 teaspoon sea salt
- 3/4 cup kamut flour
- 1/2 cup blueberries
- 1/4 cup sea moss gel (optional)
- Grapeseed oil

Directions:

1. Preheat your oven to 400 degrees F.

2. Add the flour, milk, sea salt, sea moss and agave in a bowl and mix until well integrated. Now fold in the blueberries.
3. Coat a muffin pan lightly with grapeseed oil and pour in the batter
4. Bake for 25-30 minutes
5. Enjoy!
6. Nutritional information per muffin: Calories: 144 Fat: 1.61g Carbohydrates: 26.04 Protein: 4.73g

---

Spelt Pancakes

Servings: 3

Ingredients:

- 1 cup spelt flour
- 1/4 teaspoon fine sea salt
- 2 tablespoons plant-based milk
- 1/2 cup sesame seeds
- ½ cup hemp seeds
- 1 1/2 teaspoons ground cloves
- 1/2 teaspoon agave
- 1 teaspoon coconut oil

Directions:

1. Grind the sesame seeds and hemp seeds into flour and store a quarter of the seed flour for later use (you won't need it here).
2. Now add 2 cups of the seed flour to a bowl and mix, and then add the rest of the Ingredients: except the coconut oil. You can add more milk if you need to do so to achieve the right consistency.
3. Heat a non-stick pan with coconut oil and pour a bit of the batter into the pan to make your pancake; when you see bubbles appear on top, flip once.
4. Go on with this step until you finish the pancake batter.
5. Nutritional information per (4.2 oz.) serving: Calories: 513 Carbohydrates: 49.65 g Fat: 30.69 g Protein: 18.8g

---

Teff Porridge

Servings: 2

Ingredients:

- 1/2 cup Teff grain
- Pinch of sea salt
- Blueberries (optional)
- 2 cups spring water
- Agave (optional)

Directions:

1. Bring the spring water to a boil in a saucepan. Add some sea salt and then add the teff grain (after the water boils) to the saucepan. Stir as you add, and then cover with a lid. Lower the heat and simmer for fifteen minutes.
2. Add the agave and blueberries as toppings, as desired and enjoy your porridge!
3. Nutritional information per (10 oz.) serving (excluding the optional Ingredients:): Calories: 177 Fat: 1.15g Carbohydrates: 35.29g Protein: 6.42g

---

Quinoa Breakfast

Servings: 3

Ingredients:

- 1 cup quinoa, rinsed
- 1/2 teaspoon vanilla
- 1/4 teaspoon allspice
- 1 medium apple chopped small (you can save some for garnishing)
- 1/2 cup raw walnuts, chopped
- 1 cup fresh organic blueberries
- 3 cups walnut milk
- 1 teaspoon ground cloves
- 1/2 cup raisins
- Agave to taste
- 4 tablespoons your favorite seeds
- Fresh raspberries, strawberries (optional)

Directions:

1. Add the almond milk, quinoa, allspice, ground cloves and raisins to a medium bowl and mix. Bring to a boil, place a lid on the pan and set the heat to low.
2. After five minutes, add the chopped apple while stirring and simmer for 5-7 more minutes. Stir and check for any remaining liquid. If most of it is absorbed, remove it from the heat, leave the lid on the pan and allow it to rest for about five minutes to absorb the remaining milk.
3. When that time is over, you can still simmer for 3-5 more minutes if you can still see a lot of liquid in there; just make sure to keep a close eye on it as the mixture can burn very easily if you leave it to boil dry, and then allow it to rest for five minutes.
4. Taste it for sweetness and adjust it to your desire with a dribble of agave. You may not require any extra sweetener though because the raisins and apple are naturally sweet.
5. To serve, top each bowl with favorite seeds, walnuts, the rest of the chopped apples and blueberries. You can also toss some strawberries or raspberries if you have them at hand!

6. Nutritional information per (10.2 oz.) serving: Calories: 858 Fat: 56.78g Carbohydrates: 76.49g Protein: 22.1 g

---

Spelt Chapatti

Yield: 2 chapattis

Ingredients:

- 1/3 cup spelt flour
- 2 tablespoons lukewarm water
- 1/4 teaspoon salt (maybe more to sprinkle)
- 1/2 teaspoon white sesame seeds (optional)

Directions:

1. Add the flour and salt to a mixing bowl and mix. Add the water bit by bit until you have a smooth dough.
2. You can knead using your hands until you form a smooth dough or use a kitchen machine with a knead hook if you have one. Remember that you might have to triple or at least double the amounts for the machine to work properly.
3. Cover the dough with a clean kitchen towel and give it some time to rest in the bowl for half an hour or so. Divide the dough into two and roll them out on a nicely floured surface.
4. You can sprinkle some sesame seeds and a pinch of salt over the flatbread and roll the seeds lightly into the dough using a rolling pin.
5. Get a crepe pan and heat it well (the hotter the better).
6. Place one chapatti and let it cook for 30 seconds on each side. Repeat the process with the other bit of dough.
7. When ready, serve and enjoy with your favorite curry.
8. Nutritional information per chapatti: Calories: 82 Carbohydrates: 14 g Protein: 2 g

---

Chickpea Burgers

Servings: 8 Burgers

Ingredients:

- 3 cups canned or cooked chickpeas
- 1 cup of kale, chopped
- 1 teaspoon cayenne
- 2 green onions, chopped
- Salt to taste
- 1/3 cup of dry quinoa, washed and drained
- 1/4 cup chickpea flour

- 2 teaspoons each of oregano, dill and basil
- Spring water as needed

Directions:

1. Toast the quinoa in a hot pan to cook it. Once the quinoa has separated, add two-thirds of the one cup of water to the pan and bring to a boil. Cover with a tight lid and give the quinoa fifteen minutes to cook over low flame. Turn off the heat and give it about ten minutes to sit, covered.
2. Mash the chickpeas in a large bowl. You should be expecting to have some large pieces in there for texture, but not so big, otherwise the patty will not hold. Add the cooked quinoa, chopped kale, chickpea flour, seasonings and cayenne, and add salt to taste.
3. Add water as you find necessary to make the right consistency to create the patties. Meanwhile, preheat your oven to 375 degrees F.
4. Divide the mixture into eight parts, and pat each part into a nice, round and flat patty; you can definitely make it bigger or smaller if you want.
5. Brush the baking sheet with a thin layer of oil, and then place the patties on the pan evenly. Bake in your oven for fifteen minutes and then flip to cook the other side.
6. Serve on the rye burger buns or spelt with some cherry tomatoes, onion, and zucchini slices. You can also add some avocado salsa.
7. Don't know how to make an avocado sauce?
8. It's real simple:
9. Just add jalapeno, avocado, lime juice, water, olive oil and salt in a food processor and process until smooth.
10. Add the onion and pulse. Serve as a dressing for your burger.
11. Nutritional information per Burger Calories: 145 Fat: 2.3 g Carbohydrates: 24.4 g Protein: 7.41 g

---

Alkaline Biscuits

Servings: 6 Biscuits

Ingredients:

- 1 ½ cups white spelt flour
- 7 tablespoons spring water
- ¼ cup chilled grapeseed oil or avocado oil
- 1 tablespoon agave
- 1 teaspoon sea salt

Directions:

1. Combine the flour and sea salt and stir until they are well integrated.
2. Add all the wet Ingredients: into the mixture and stir again until they are all well combined. Finish mixing the dough with your hand.

3. To form the biscuits, break the dough apart into six pieces or roll it out and cut the pieces out with a cutter.
4. Grease the cookware lightly with the oil you are using. Put the biscuit pieces on the cookie sheet and bake for 11-13 minutes at 350 degrees, and then place them under the broiler for 1 or 2 more minutes to brown just lightly.
5. Remove them from the pan and allow them to cool for a little while. Serve warm with agave.
6. Nutritional information per Biscuit: Calories: 153 Fat: 1.07g Carbohydrates: 32.05g Protein: 6.4

Portobello Mushroom Patties

Servings: 1 Patty

Ingredients:

- 2 portobello mushrooms
- 1/4 teaspoon oregano (dry/ fresh)
- 1/4 cup of culantro
- 2 teaspoons onion powder (or red onion)
- 1/2 cup bell peppers (red /green)
- 1 pinch of cayenne pepper
- 1/4 teaspoon sea salt, to taste
- 1/4 cup of flour (spelt, rye)

Directions:

1. Soak the mushrooms in water for one minute. When ready, remove them, and put them in a food processor, along with bell peppers and culantro (you can dice up the mushrooms and peppers if you don't have a food processor) and process them.
2. Now add the flour and the seasonings and mix well to form a patty. Put the patty in a heated pan with two tablespoons of oil and fry on both sides until ready.
3. Nutritional information per Patty Calories: 188 Fat: 1.62g Carbohydrates: 39.01 g Protein: 11.4 g

Spelt Waffles

Servings: 4

Ingredients:

- 2 ½ cups spelt flour
- ½ teaspoon sea salt
- 1 cup spring water
- 3 tablespoons date sugar
- 1 ½ cups hemp milk
- 3 tablespoons hemp seed oil

Directions:

1. Add the sugar, flour and salt to a mixing bowl and whisk them together. Add the water, oil and milk and stir until well integrated, keeping in mind that a thick batter is most ideal for waffles.
2. Preheat the waffle maker on desired setting (you can set to 3) and only brush with oil once for all the waffles.
3. When your waffle maker is ready, add ½ cup of the batter to the center of the machine and cook until ready.
4. Repeat the process with the rest of the batter.
5. Serve either warm or cold with a drizzle of agave cactus syrup on top.
6. Nutritional information per (9.5 oz.) serving: Calories: 404 Fat: 14.9 g Carbohydrates: 60.9 g Protein: 11.2 g

---

Spelt Porridge

Servings: 1 Serving

Ingredients:

- 1 cup filtered water
- 1/4 teaspoon alcohol free vanilla
- 1/3 cup thin-flaked spelt
- Agave syrup to taste
- 2-3 tablespoons dried cherries
- Toppings
- Walnuts, fresh berries, seeds, almond or hemp milk

Directions:

1. Add all the Ingredients: into a pan and simmer over medium heat for 3-4 minutes, and then pour into a medium bowl.
2. Pour some walnut milk and add your favorite toppings.
3. Nutritional information per (11.8 oz.) serving Calories: 219 Fat: 1.5 g Carbohydrates: 44.6 g Protein: 8.66g

---

Chickpea Pancakes

Servings: 6 pancakes

Ingredients:

- 3/4 cup of spelt flour
- 1 cup of hemp milk
- 2 tablespoons of agave
- Grapeseed oil
- 1/4 cup of chickpea flour
- 2 tablespoons of sea moss gel

- 1/8 teaspoon of sea salt

Directions:

1. Add the chickpea flour and spelt to a large mixing bowl and mix well. Add the sea moss, hemp milk, sea salt and agave and mix some more.
2. Oil your skillet with the grape-seed oil before you pour in the batter depending on the size you want.
3. Flip each pancake when it turns golden brown on both sides.
4. Add toppings like fruit or agave and enjoy.
5. Nutritional information per (2-pancake) serving   Calories: 203 Fat: 3.73g Carbohydrates: 35.94g Protein: 8.95g

---

Quinoa Porridge

Servings: 4

Ingredients:

- 1 cup of dry quinoa
- 1/2 teaspoon cayenne
- 1/2 cup of coconut cream or milk (this depends on how creamy you'd love it to be)
- 1 grated apple
- 2 cups of water
- 1/2 lime skin grated
- Cloves, ground (optional)
- Half a handful of assorted nuts and seeds (choose your favorite, but alkaline-friendly)

Directions:

1. First, prepare the quinoa according to the instructions on the packet. When it is well cooked, drain it and put it back in the saucepan and add in the cloves and cayenne while stirring (if you prepared them in a pestle and mortar) and then pour in the coconut milk or cream.
2. When ready, add the grated apple (if using) – this should come at the very end.
3. Allow the apple to warm through and then serve your porridge. Add the grated lime rind onto the top and add a few nuts and seeds (sesame seeds would be great here).
4. Nutritional information per (8.5 oz.) serving Calories: 251 Fat: 9.8 g Carbohydrates: 35 g Protein: 6.8 g

Spelt & Rye Bread

Servings: 1 loaf

Ingredients:

- 2 cups rye flour
- ½ teaspoons of Dr. Sebi bromide plus powder (you can also use 2 tablespoons sea moss)
- 2 cups hemp milk
- Sesame seeds (optional)
- 2 cups spelt flour
- 1 teaspoon sea salt
- 2 tablespoons agave

Note:

- If you want, you can also use four cups of spelt flour particularly if you don't love rye's taste- or vice versa.
- If you choose to use the sea moss, keep it in mind that the batter might get stickier

Directions:

1. Preheat your oven to 350 degrees F. Meanwhile, sift the flour into a bowl.
2. Add the dry Ingredients: into the bowl with the flour and mix.
3. Add the agave and mix for five or so minutes. Grease and flour your loaf pan by coating it lightly with the grapeseed oil and flour. Add the dough into the pan and level it out.
4. Brush the grapeseed oil over the bread and sprinkle the sesame seeds on top to your liking.
5. Bake the bread in your oven for 60 minutes at 350 degrees F.
6. Allow it to set for 20 minutes, or until it cools.
7. Enjoy a slice or two with your favorite herbal tea.
8. Nutritional Information for the (2 lb.) Loaf Calories: 2222 Fat: 29.21 g Carbohydrates: 426 g Protein: 88.97 g

---

Apple-Nut Porridge

Servings: 1 serving

Ingredients:

- 2 tablespoons coarsely chopped walnuts
- 2 coarsely chopped dried white figs
- 1 teaspoon dried goji berries
- 1 peeled Granny Smith apple, cored and coarsely chopped
- 1/2 teaspoon ground sesame seeds
- 1/4 teaspoon chopped fresh ginger

Directions:

1. Grind the nuts in a food processor and then add the figs, ginger and apple; process until chunky and transfer the porridge to a bowl. Top with ground seeds and goji berries.
2. Nutritional information per (7 oz.) serving: Calories: 277 Fat: 10 g Carbohydrates: 48g Protein: 5.5g

---

Brazil Nut Banana Bread

Servings: 1 (4lb.) Loaf

Ingredients:

- 2 cups sprouted spelt flour
- 6 tablespoons sesame seeds
- 1 ½ teaspoons ground cloves
- 1 cup agave syrup
- 4 burro bananas
- 1/4 cup walnut butter
- 1 cup quinoa flour
- 1/2 teaspoon fine sea salt
- 2/3 cup coconut oil
- 2 teaspoons vanilla extract
- 1 cup plain nut milk (from your favorite nuts)
- 10 Brazil nuts

Directions:

1. Mix the seeds, flour, cloves and sea salt in a large mixing bowl and set aside.
2. Add the nut milk, coconut oil (melt it first) and agave syrup to a blender and blend until smooth. Add the bananas (cut into pieces) and pulse for 10-20 more seconds to combine. Add the wet mixture into the dry mixture and using a spatula, fold together until they just mix.
3. Line a loaf pan (9x5 inches) with parchment paper and add the banana bread mixture into the pan. Chop the Brazil nuts and sprinkle on the top of the loaf evenly. You can also mix these into the batter directly.
4. Let the loaf bake for one hour and ten minutes (after one hour, check with a knife to see whether it is ready because each oven is always different).
5. Remove from the pan and allow it to cool on a wire rack once ready. Slice it and serve; store the leftovers in an airtight container.
6. This loaf is best eaten within four days.
7. Nutritional information for the (4 lb.) loaf: Calories: 5330 Fat: 250g Carbohydrates: 741g Protein: 98g

Vegan Muffins

Servings: 9 muffins

Ingredients:

- 1 cup hemp milk, coconut milk, walnut milk or quinoa milk
- 3/4 cup kamut flour
- 1/3 cup agave nectar
- 1/2 teaspoon sea salt
- 3/4 cup teff flour
- 2 apples (peeled and chopped)
- 1/4 cup sea moss gel
- 1 teaspoon ground cloves

Directions:

1. Preheat your oven to 400 degrees F. Meanwhile, add all the dry Ingredients: to a mixing bowl and combine.
2. Add the milk, sea moss gel and agave nectar into the mixture and then fold the apples into it.
3. Grease a muffin tin and add the batter; bake for about 30 minutes or when you insert a toothpick in the center of one muffin, it should come out clean.
4. Finally, let the muffins cool and remove them from the pan.
5. Serve and enjoy!
6. Note:
7. Given that, we did not add any leavening to our recipe; your muffins will come out slightly dense. However, that is common to nearly all alkaline vegan baked foods.
8. Nutritional information per muffin: Calories: 136 Fat: 1.49g Carbohydrates: 27.07g Protein: 4.21g

---

Quinoa Bowl

Servings: 4

Ingredients:

- 3/4 cup dry quinoa
- 3/4 cup canned coconut milk
- 1 date, chopped
- Pinch of salt
- 1 1/2 cups water
- 1/2 cup hemp milk
- 2 teaspoons ground cloves
- 2 teaspoons vanilla extract
- Any desired toppings (such as burro banana, coconut flakes, blueberries or walnuts)

Directions:

1. Add the water and quinoa to a medium saucepan and bring to a boil. Lower the heat and cook covered for 13-15 minutes, until the quinoa becomes fluffy.
2. While the heat is still low, add the coconut milk, hemp milk, salt, sweetener and the seasonings. Stir well to combine, and cook until most of the milk has been absorbed (by the quinoa), but is still pourable. You can add more milk as needed.
3. Pour a bit of it into a bowl and add more of the milk along with the toppings.
4. Nutritional information per (7 oz.) serving Calories: 178 Fat: 4.45g Carbohydrates: 26. 7g Protein: 7.4 g

---

Quinoa & Apple Breakfast

Servings: 1 Serving

Ingredients:

- ½ cup of quinoa
- ½ lemon
- 1 apple
- 1 cup water
- Cayenne or any alkaline spice of your choice

Directions:

1. Rinse the quinoa in a sieve, add water and then bring to a boil; simmer for 15 minutes.
2. As the 15 minutes ends, grate the apple and add to the quinoa, and allow it to cook for 30 more seconds. Similarly, grate the lemon zest, add, and then squeeze in a bit of lemon to taste.
3. To serve, sprinkle your spice and enjoy.
4. Nutritional information per (10 oz.) serving: Calories: 413 Fat: 5.5g Carbohydrates: 81g Protein: 12.5g

---

Breakfast Porridge

Servings: 6

Ingredients:

- 1/4 cup walnuts
- 1 cup and 6 tablespoons hemp milk
- 1 cup fonio grains
- 2 cups water
- 4 dates, pitted and chopped
- 1/2 cup raisins
- 1/2 cup fresh blueberries
- 6 tablespoons shredded coconut

Directions:

1. Toast the nuts in a skillet over medium-low heat for five minutes. Chop them into large pieces and set aside.
2. Add the fonio and water to a medium-sized saucepan and stir to remove any lumps. Add the dates and bring to a boil, making sure to stir often as you crush the pieces of dates. When you notice the dates starting to dissolve, lower the heat to a simmer and add the raisins and milk.
3. Keep simmering while stirring often until all the liquid has been absorbed; this should take around 8 minutes.
4. To serve, pour the porridge into six bowls and top with the blueberries, toasted nuts, the spice and 6 tablespoons of milk.
5. Nutritional information per (7 oz.) serving: Calories: 210 Fat: 6.37g Carbohydrates: 32.96g Protein: 6.9g

---

Fonio Cereal

Servings: 4

Ingredients:

- 1 ½ cups fonio
- ½ teaspoon salt
- Agave to sweeten (optional)
- 4 ½ cups hemp milk
- Fruit of choice (optional)

Directions:

1. Wash the fonio and add it to a medium-sized pot. Add in the milk and bring to a simmer on low heat, stirring often for half an hour. The fonio grains should be tender, having absorbed the milk.
2. When the grains become tender, add the salt, stir well and serve warm. You may serve the fonio with fruit toppings or even nuts and agave.
3. Nutritional information per (9.7 oz.) serving: Calories: 128.9 Fat: 1.8 g Carbohydrates: 9.97 g Protein: 4.55g

Chapter 5. Lunch

Tomato & Greens Salad

Preparation time: 15 minutes.

Servings: 4

Ingredients:

- 6 cups fresh baby greens
- 2 cups cherry tomatoes
- 2 scallions, chopped
- 2 tbsp extra-virgin olive oil
- 2 tbsp fresh orange juice
- 1 tbsp fresh lemon juice

Directions:

1. Place all the Ingredients: in a large bowl and toss to coat well.
2. Cover the bowl and refrigerate for about 6-8 hours.
3. Remove from the refrigerator and toss well before serving.

Nutrition: Calories 88; Total Fat 7.2 g; Saturated Fat 1.1 g; Cholesterol 0 mg; Sodium 11 mg; Total Carbs 5.9 g; Fiber 1.8 g; Sugar 3.8 g; Protein 1.5 g;

Strawberry & Apple Salad

Preparation time: 15 minutes.

Servings: 4

Ingredients:

- For Salad:
- 4 cups mixed lettuce, torn
- 2 apples, cored and sliced
- 1 cup fresh strawberries, hulled and sliced
- ¼ cup pecans, chopped
- For Dressing:
- 3 tbsp apple cider vinegar
- 3 tbsp olive oil
- 1 tbsp agave nectar
- 1 tsp poppy seeds

Directions:

1. For the salad, place all the Ingredients: in a large bowl and mix well.
2. For the dressing, place all the Ingredients: in a bowl and beat until well combined.
3. Pour the dressing over the salad and toss it all to coat well.
4. Serve immediately.

Nutrition: Calories 244; Total Fat 16.9 g; Saturated Fat 2.1 g; Cholesterol 0 mg; Sodium 5 mg; Total Carbs 25.2 g; Fiber 5 g; Sugar 18.1 g; Protein 1.8 g

---

Cauliflower Soup

Preparation time: 15 minutes

Cooking time: 30 minutes.

Servings: 4

Ingredients:

- 2 tbsp olive oil
- 1 yellow onion, chopped
- 2 carrots, peeled and chopped
- 2 garlic cloves, minced
- 1 Serrano pepper, chopped finely
- 2 celery stalks, chopped
- 1 tsp ground turmeric
- 1 tsp ground coriander
- 1 tsp ground cumin
- ¼ tsp red pepper flakes, crushed
- 1 head cauliflower, chopped
- 4 cups homemade vegetable broth
- 1 cup unsweetened coconut milk
- Sea salt and freshly ground black pepper, to taste
- 2 tbsp fresh chives, chopped finely

Directions:

1. Heat the oil over medium heat in a large soup pan and sauté the onion, carrot, and celery for about 4-6 minutes.
2. Add the garlic, Serrano pepper, and spices and sauté for about 1 minute.
3. Add the cauliflower and cook for about 5 minutes, stirring occasionally.
4. Add the broth and coconut milk and bring to a boil over medium-high heat.
5. Reduce the heat to low and simmer for about 15 minutes.
6. Season the soup with the salt and black pepper and remove it from the heat.
7. With an immersion blender, blend the soup until smooth.
8. Serve hot and garnish with chives.

Nutrition: Calories 285; Total Fat 23 g; Saturated Fat 14.1 g; Cholesterol 0 mg; Sodium 881 mg; Total Carbs 14.9 g; Fiber 4.8 g; Sugar 7.2 g; Protein 4.5 g

Tomato Soup

Preparation time: 15 minutes

Cooking time: 45 minutes. Total time: 1 hour

Servings: 4

Ingredients:

- 2 tbsp coconut oil
- 2 carrots, chopped roughly
- 1 large white onion, chopped roughly
- 3 garlic cloves, minced
- 5 large tomatoes, chopped roughly
- 1 tbsp homemade tomato paste
- 3 cups homemade vegetable broth
- ¼ cup fresh basil, chopped
- ¼ cup unsweetened coconut milk
- Sea salt and freshly ground black pepper, to taste

Directions:

1. Melt the coconut oil in a large soup pan over medium heat and cook the carrot and onion for about 10 minutes, stirring frequently.
2. Add the garlic and sauté for about 1-2 minutes.
3. Stir in the tomatoes, tomato paste, basil, broth, salt and black pepper and bring to a boil.
4. Reduce the heat to low and simmer uncovered for about 30 minutes.
5. Stir in the coconut milk and remove from the heat.
6. With an immersion blender, blend the soup until smooth.
7. Serve hot.

Nutrition: Calories 197; Total Fat 12 g; Saturated Fat 9.4 g; Cholesterol 0 mg; Sodium 671 mg; Total Carbs 18.4 g; Fiber 4.8 g; Sugar 10.6 g; Protein 7 g

---

Garlicky Broccoli

Preparation time: 10 minutes

Cooking time: 8 minutes.

Servings: 2

Ingredients:

- 1 tbsp extra-virgin olive oil
- 3-4 garlic cloves, minced
- 2 cups broccoli florets
- 2 tbsp tamari

Directions:

1. Heat the oil over medium heat in a large skillet and sauté the garlic for about 1 minute.
2. Add the broccoli and stir fry for about 2 minutes.
3. Stir in the tamari and stir fry for about 4-5 minutes or until desired doneness.
4. Remove from the heat and serve hot.

Nutrition: Calories 109; Total Fat 7.3 g; Saturated Fat 1 g; Cholesterol 0 mg; Sodium 1,000 mg; Total Carbs 8.5 g; Fiber 2.6 g; Sugar 1.9 g; Protein 4.7 g

---

Curried Okra

Preparation time: 10 minutes

Cooking time: 15 minutes.

Servings: 3

Ingredients:

- 1 tbsp olive oil
- ½ tsp cumin seeds
- ¾ lb okra pods, trimmed and cut into 2-inch pieces
- ½ tsp curry powder
- ½ tsp red chili powder
- 1 tsp ground coriander
- Sea salt and freshly ground black pepper, to taste

Directions:

1. Heat the oil in a large skillet over medium heat
2. For about 30 seconds, sauté the cumin seeds
3. Add the okra and stir fry for about 1-1½ minutes.
4. Reduce the heat to low and cook covered for about 6-8 minutes stirring occasionally.
5. Add the curry powder, red chili, and coriander and stir to combine.
6. Increase the heat to medium and cook uncovered for about 2-3 minutes more.
7. Season with the salt and pepper and remove from the heat.
8. Serve hot.

Nutrition: Calories 89; Total Fat 5.1 g; Saturated Fat 0.7 g; Cholesterol 0 mg; Sodium 91 mg; Total Carbs 9 g; Fiber 3.9 g; Sugar 1.7 g; Protein 2.3 g

Mushroom Curry

Preparation time: 20 minutes

Cooking time: 20 minutes.

Servings: 4

Ingredients:

- 2 cup tomatoes, chopped
- 1 green chili, chopped
- 1 tsp fresh ginger, chopped
- 2 tbsp olive oil
- ½ tsp cumin seeds
- ¼ tsp ground coriander
- ¼ tsp ground turmeric
- ¼ tsp red chili powder
- 2 cups fresh shiitake mushrooms, sliced
- 2 cups fresh button mushrooms, sliced
- 1¼ cups water
- ¼ cup unsweetened coconut milk
- Sea salt and freshly ground black pepper, to taste

Directions:

1. In a food processor, add the tomatoes, green chili and ginger and pulse until a smooth paste forms.
2. Heat the oil in a pan over medium heat.
3. For about 1 minute, sauté the cumin seeds.
4. Add the spices and sauté for about 1 minute.
5. Add the tomato mixture and cook for about 5 minutes.
6. Stir in the mushrooms, water, and coconut milk and bring to a boil.
7. Cook for about 10-12 minutes, stirring occasionally.
8. Season with the salt and black pepper and remove from the heat.
9. Serve hot.

Nutrition: Calories 161; Total Fat 11.2 g; Saturated Fat 4.3 g; Cholesterol 0 mg; Sodium 224 mg; Total Carbs 16.1 g; Fiber 3.5 g; Sugar 6.1 g; Protein 3.5 g

---

Glazed Brussels Sprouts

Preparation time: 15 minutes

Cooking time: 15 minutes.

Servings: 3

Ingredients:

- 3 cups Brussels sprouts, trimmed and halved
- Sea salt, to taste
- 2 tsp coconut oil, melted
- For Orange Glaze:
- 1 tsp coconut oil
- 2 small shallots, sliced thinly

- 2 tsp fresh orange zest, grated finely
- ¼ tsp ground ginger
- 2/3 cup fresh orange juice
- 1 tsp sambal oelek (raw chili paste)
- 2 tbsp coconut aminos
- 1 tsp tapioca starch
- Sea salt, to taste

Directions:

1. Preheat the oven to 400 degrees F. Line a roasting pan with parchment paper.
2. In a bowl, add Brussels sprouts, a little salt, and oil and toss to coat well.
3. Transfer the mixture into the prepared roasting pan.
4. Roast for about 10-15 minutes, flipping once halfway through.
5. Meanwhile, prepare the glaze.
6. In a skillet, melt the coconut oil over medium heat and sauté the shallots for about 5 minutes.
7. Add the orange zest and sauté for about 1 minute.
8. Stir in ginger, orange juice, sambal oelek, and coconut aminos and cook for about 5 minutes.
9. Slowly, add the tapioca starch, beating continuously.
10. Cook for about 2-3 minutes more, stirring frequently.
11. Stir in the salt and remove from the heat.
12. Transfer the roasted Brussels sprouts to a serving plate. Top with orange glaze evenly.
13. Serve immediately garnished with scallions.

Nutrition: Calories 132; Total Fat 5 g; Saturated Fat 4 g; Cholesterol 0 mg; Sodium 124 mg; Total Carbs 20.6 g; Fiber 4.4 g; Sugar 8.2 g; Protein 3.8 g

Sautéed Mushrooms

Preparation time: 15 minutes

Cooking time: 16 minutes.

Servings: 2

Ingredients:

- 2 tbsp olive oil
- ½ tsp cumin seeds, crushed lightly
- 2 medium onions, sliced thinly
- ¾ lb fresh mushrooms, chopped
- Sea salt and freshly ground black pepper, to taste

Directions:

1. Heat the oil in a skillet over medium heat

2. For about 1 minute, sauté the cumin seeds.
3. Add the onion and sauté for about 4-5 minutes.
4. Add the mushrooms and sauté for about 5-7 minutes.
5. Add the salt and black pepper and sauté for about 2-3 minutes.
6. Remove from the heat and serve hot.

Nutrition: Calories 202; Total Fat 14.7 g; Saturated Fat 2 g; Cholesterol 0 mg; Sodium 132 mg; Total Carbs 16.1 g; Fiber 4.1 g; Sugar 7.6 g; Protein 66 g

---

Sweet & Sour Kale

Preparation time: 10 minutes

Cooking time: 20 minutes.

Servings: 4

Ingredients:

- 1 tbsp extra-virgin olive oil
- 1 lemon, seeded sliced thinly
- 1 onion, chopped
- 3 garlic cloves, minced
- 2 lb fresh kale, tough ribs removed and chopped
- ½ cup scallions, chopped
- 1 tbsp agave nectar
- Sea salt and freshly ground black pepper, to taste

Directions:

1. In a large skillet, heat oil over medium heat and cook the lemon slices for about 5 minutes.
2. With a slotted spoon, remove the lemon slices.
3. In the same skillet, add the onion and garlic and sauté for about 5 minutes.
4. Add the kale, scallions, agave nectar, salt, and black pepper and cook for about 8-10 minutes, stirring occasionally.
5. Remove from the heat and serve hot.

Nutrition: Calories 175; Total Fat 3.6 g; Saturated Fat 0.5 g; Cholesterol 0 mg; Sodium 160 mg; Total Carbs 31.9 g; Fiber 4.6 g; Sugar 5.2 g; Protein 7.4 g

Nutty Brussels Sprouts

Preparation time: 15 minutes

Cooking time: 15 minutes

Servings: 2

Ingredients:

- ½ pound Brussels sprouts, halved
- 1 tablespoon olive oil
- 2 garlic cloves, minced
- ½ teaspoon red pepper flakes, crushed
- Sea salt and freshly ground black pepper, to taste
- 1 tablespoon fresh lemon juice
- 1 tablespoon pine nuts

Directions:

1. Arrange a steamer basket in a large pan of boiling water.
2. Place the Brussels sprouts in steamer basket and steam, covered for about 6-8 minutes.
3. Drain the Brussels sprouts well.
4. In a large skillet, heat the oil over medium heat and sauté the garlic and red pepper flakes for about 40 seconds.
5. Stir in the Brussels sprouts, salt, and black pepper and sauté for about 4-5 minutes.
6. Stir in lemon juice and sauté for about 1 minute more.
7. Stir in the pine nuts and remove from the heat.
8. Serve hot.

Nutrition: Calories 146 Total Fat 10.5 g Saturated Fat 1.4 g Cholesterol 0 mg Sodium 148 mg Total Carbs 12.3 g Fiber 4.6 g Sugar 2.8 g Protein 4.8 g

Roasted Butternut Squash

Preparation time: 15 minutes

Cooking time: 45 minutes

Servings: 6

Ingredients:

- 8 cups butternut squash, peeled, seeded, and cubed
- 2 tablespoons melted almond butter
- ½ teaspoon ground cinnamon
- ½ teaspoon ground cumin
- ¼ teaspoon red pepper flakes
- Sea salt, to taste

Directions:

1. Preheat oven to 425 degrees F. Arrange pieces of foil on 2 baking sheets.
2. In a large bowl, add all the Ingredients: and toss to coat well.
3. Arrange the squash pieces onto the prepared baking sheets in a single layer.
4. Roast for about 40-45 minutes.
5. Remove from the oven and serve.

Nutrition: Calories 118 Total Fat 3.2 g Saturated Fat 0.3 g Cholesterol 0 mg Sodium 47 mg Total Carbs 23.1 g Fiber 4.4 g Sugar 4.4 g Protein 3.1 g

---

Broccoli with Bell Pepper

Preparation time: 15 minutes

Cooking time: 10 minutes

Servings: 4

Ingredients:

- 2 tablespoons olive oil
- 4 garlic cloves, minced
- 1 large white onion, sliced
- 2 cups small broccoli florets
- 3 red bell peppers, seeded and sliced
- ¼ cup homemade vegetable broth
- Sea salt and freshly ground black pepper, to taste

Directions:

1. In a large skillet, heat the oil over medium heat and sauté the garlic for about 1 minute.
2. Add the onion, broccoli, and bell peppers and stir fry for about 5 minutes.
3. Add the broth and stir fry for about 4 minutes more.
4. Serve hot.

Nutrition: Calories 126 Total Fat 7.5 g Saturated Fat 1 g Cholesterol 0 mg Sodium 125 mg Total Carbs 14.3 g Fiber 2.3 g Sugar 6.9 g Protein 3.1 g

Tamari Shrimp

Preparation time: 15 minutes

Cooking time: 6 minutes

Servings: 2

Ingredients:

- 1 tablespoon olive oil
- 2 garlic cloves, minced
- ½ pound raw jumbo shrimp, peeled and deveined
- 2 tablespoons tamari
- Freshly ground black pepper, to taste

Directions:

1. In a large skillet, heat the oil over medium heat and sauté the garlic for about 1 minute.
2. Stir in the shrimp, tamari and black pepper and cook for about 4-5 minutes or until done completely.
3. Serve hot.

Nutrition: Calories 156 Total Fat 7 g Saturated Fat 1 g Cholesterol 233 mg Sodium 2000 mg Total Carbs 2 g Fiber 0.2 g Sugar 2.4 g Protein 22.3 g

---

Veggie Kebabs

Preparation time: 20 minutes

Cooking time: 10 minutes

Servings: 4

Ingredients:

- For Marinade:
- 2 garlic cloves, minced
- 2 teaspoons fresh basil, minced
- 2 teaspoons fresh oregano, minced
- ½ teaspoon cayenne pepper
- Sea salt and freshly ground black pepper, to taste
- 2 tablespoons fresh lemon juice
- 2 tablespoons olive oil
- For Veggies:
- 2 large zucchinis, cut into thick slices
- 8 large button mushrooms, quartered
- 1 yellow bell pepper, seeded and cubed
- 1 red bell pepper, seeded and cubed

Directions:

1. For marinade: in a large bowl, add all the Ingredients: and mix until well combined.
2. Add the vegetables to the marinade and toss to coat well.
3. Cover and refrigerate to marinate the veggies for at least 6-8 hours.
4. In a large bowl of the water, soak the wooden skewers for at least 30 minutes.
5. Preheat the grill to medium-high heat. Generously grease the grill grate.
6. Remove the vegetables from the bowl and discard the marinade.
7. Thread the vegetables onto the pre-soaked wooden skewers, starting with the zucchini, mushrooms and bell peppers.
8. Grill for about 8-10 minutes or until done completely, flipping occasionally.

Nutrition: Calories 122 Total Fat 7.8 g Saturated Fat 1.2 g Cholesterol 0 mg Sodium 81 mg Total Carbs 12.7 g Fiber 3.5 g Sugar 6.8g Protein 4.3 g

---

Sprout Onion Fry

Preparation time: 5 minutes

Cooking time: 10 minutes

Servings: 04

Ingredients:

- 2½ pounds Brussels sprouts, trimmed4 slices bacon, cut into 1-inch pieces
- 1 tablespoon extra-virgin coconut oil
- 1 tomato, chopped
- 1 onion, chopped
- 4 sprigs thyme or savory, divided
- 1 teaspoon Celtic sea salt, iodine free
- Freshly ground pepper to taste
- 2 teaspoons lemon juice (optional)

Directions:

1. Add sprouts to the boiling water in a stockpot.
2. Let them cook for about3 to 5 minutes.
3. Drain and set them aside.
4. Saute onions in a greased skillet for 4 minutes.
5. Stir in salt, pepper, and thyme
6. Add drained sprouts to the skillet and stir cook for 3 minutes.
7. Remove and discard the herb sprigs.
8. Serve warm with lemon juice and chopped spring onion on top.

Nutrition: Calories 383 Total Fat 5.3 g Saturated Fat 3.9 g Cholesterol 135 mg Sodium 487 mg Total Carbs 76.8 g Fibre 0.1g Sugar 0 g Protein 27.7 g

Southwest Stuffed Sweet Potatoes

Ingredients:

- Sliced avocado (1)
- Pinch of cumin
- Pinch of dried red chili flakes
- Spinach (3 c.)
- Sliced shallot (1)
- Black beans (.5 c.)
- Coconut oil (2 Tbsp.)
- Sweet potatoes
- The dressing
- Pepper and salt
- Minced cilantro (1 handful)
- Cumin (1 tsp.)
- Juiced lime (1)
- Olive oil (3 Tbsp.)

Directions:

1. Turn on the oven and give it time to heat up to 400 degrees. Clean the sweet potatoes and pierce a few times with a fork.
2. Add some parchment paper to a baking tray and set the sweet potatoes on top. Add to the oven to bake.
3. After 50 minutes, the potatoes should be soft. Take them out of the oven and give them time to cool.
4. In the meantime, take out a skillet and add in the coconut oil along with the black beans and the shallot.
5. Cook these for a few minutes before adding in the cumin, chili flakes, and spinach, stirring around to mix well.
6. Finally, take out a small bowl and whisk the Ingredients: for the dressing together well.
7. Slice the sweet potatoes down the middle before stuffing with the mixture of black beans that you made.
8. Top with some of the slices of avocado along with some of the dressing drizzled on them before serving.

Zoodles with Cream Sauce

Ingredients:

- Toasted pepitas (2 Tbsp.)
- Pepper (.5 tsp.)
- Salt (1 tsp.)
- Minced cilantro (2 Tbsp.)
- Water (1 Tbsp.)
- Juiced lemon (.5)
- Olive oil (2 Tbsp.)
- Pitted avocado (1)
- Spiralized zucchini (1)
- Coconut oil (1 Tbsp.)

Directions:

1. Add some coconut oil to melt on a skillet before adding in the zucchini noodles. Cook for 5 minutes before turning the heat off.
2. Take out a blender and combine together the pepper, salt, a tablespoon of cilantro, water, lemon juice, oil, and avocado. Mix well and cook to make creamy.
3. Add the sauce to the skillet with your noodles and toss to combine. Move over to a serving bowl and top with the rest of the cilantro and the toasted pepitas before serving.

Rainbow Pad Thai

Ingredients:

- Diced avocado (1)
- Chopped cilantro (1 c.)
- Shredded daikon radish (1 c.)
- Chopped broccoli (1 c.)
- Shredded red cabbage (1 c.)
- Sliced scallions (3)
- Shredded carrots (2)
- Spiralized zucchini (3)
- For the dressing
- Minced ginger (1 tsp.)
- Minced garlic clove (1)
- Sesame oil (1 tsp.)
- Tahini (.25 c.)
- Juiced lime (1)

Directions:

1. Add the Ingredients: for the Pad Thai, except for the avocado, into a big bowl and toss around.
2. Whisk together all of the Ingredients: that you have for the dressing until they are creamy and combined.
3. Top the vegetables with the diced avocado and drizzle the dressing on top before serving.

Lentils and Greens

Ingredients:

- Avocado (1)
- Crushed almonds (1 tsp.)
- Crushed black pepper (1 tsp.)
- Salt (1 tsp.)
- Arugula (1 c.)
- Brown or green lentils (.5 c.)
- Cooked wild rice (1 c.)
- Juiced lemon (.5)
- Diced carrot (1)
- Broccoli florets (.5 c.)

- Sliced pak choi (.5 c.)
- Vegetable broth (.25 c.)

How to make:

1. Add the vegetable broth to a skillet on medium heat. Give it some time to start simmering before adding in the lemon juice, carrot, broccoli, and pak choi.
2. After 5 minutes, turn the heat off the stove and stir in the almonds, pepper, salt, arugula, lentils, and wild rice.
3. Move this mixture over to plates and top with some avocado slices before serving.

Sesame Greens Dish

Ingredients:

- Sesame seeds (1 tsp.)
- Juiced lemon (.5)
- Tamari sauce (2 Tbsp.)
- Minced garlic clove (1)
- Diced red bell pepper (.5 c.)
- Finely chopped broccoli florets (2 c.)
- Cubed tofu (8 oz.)
- Olive oil (2 Tbsp.)
- Sesame oil, toasted (1.5 Tbsp.)

Directions:

1. Heat up half a tablespoon of sesame oil and a tablespoon of olive oil in a pan. Add in the tofu and let it cook for a bit.
2. After ten minutes, take the tofu out and add in a bit more of the two oils.
3. Stir in the garlic, red bell pepper, and broccoli until they have time to soften a bit. Add in the tofu and stir in the lemon juice and the soy sauce as well.
4. Top this dish with some sesame seeds before serving.

Sweet Spinach Salad

Ingredients:

- Crushed black pepper (1 tsp.)
- Salt (1 tsp.)
- Nutmeg (1 tsp.)
- Cinnamon (1 tsp.)
- Chopped spinach (4 c.)
- Chopped parsley (2 Tbsp.)
- Chopped walnuts (.25 c.)
- Raisins (.25 c.)
- Sliced apple (.5 c.)
- Yogurt (.5 c.)
- Lime juice (1 tbsp.)
- Shredded carrots (.75 c.)

Directions:

1. To start this recipe, bring out a big bowl and combine all of the Ingredients: together.
2. Add the bowl to the fridge to chill for about ten minutes before serving.

Steamed Green Bowl

Ingredients:

- Chopped cilantro (2 Tbsp.)
- Salt (1 tsp.)
- Sliced green onions (2)
- Ground cashews (1 c.)
- Coconut milk (2 c.)
- Green peas (.5 c.)
- Sliced zucchini (1)
- Broccoli head (1)
- Grated ginger (1-inch piece)
- Turmeric (1 tsp.)
- Minced garlic clove (1)
- Sliced onion (1)
- Coconut oil (1 Tbsp.)

Directions:

1. Heat up some coconut oil in a pan and when it is warm, add in the ginger, turmeric, garlic, and onion.
2. After five minutes of cooking, add in the coconut milk, peas, zucchini, and broccoli to this mixture.
3. Let the Ingredients: come to a boil before reducing the heat down and simmering this for a bit.
4. After another 15 minutes, stir in the cilantro, salt, green onions, and cashews before serving.

Vegetable and Berry Salad

Ingredients:

- Raspberries (.5 c.)
- Sliced tangerine (.5)
- Alfalfa sprouts (1 c.)
- Shredded red cabbage (.5 head)
- Juiced lemon 1)
- Olive oil (3 Tbsp.)
- Diced cucumber (1)
- Avocado (1)
- Sliced shallot (1)
- Sliced kale (4 leaves)
- Chopped parsley (1 Tbsp.)
- Sliced red bell pepper (.5)
- Shredded carrot (1)
- Crushed almonds (1 Tbsp.)
- Pumpkin seeds (2 Tbsp.)

Directions:

1. Take out a large bowl and add in all of the Ingredients: to it.
2. Toss well to combine before topping the fruits and vegetables with some lemon juice and some oil.
3. Serve this right away.

Quinoa and Carrot Bowl

Ingredients:

- Sliced green onions (2 Tbsp.)
- Black sesame seeds (2 Tbsp.)
- Salt (.25 tsp.)
- Chopped parsley (3 Tbsp.)
- Juiced lemon (.5)
- Cooked quinoa (2 c.)
- Sliced fennel bulb (1)
- Carrots, chopped (1 bunch)
- Olive oil (1 Tbsp.)
- Miso (1 Tbsp.)
- Water (1 c.)

Directions:

1. Whisk together the miso and the water in a bowl. Then take out a skillet and heat up some oil inside.
2. When the oil is warm, add in the fennel bulb and carrots and cook for a few minutes, flipping over when three minutes have passed.
3. Add the water and miso mixture to the pan and reduce the heat down to a low. Cook with the lid on for a bit. This will take 20 minutes.
4. While this mixture is cooking, combine together the quinoa with the parsley, lemon juice, and salt in a bowl.
5. When the carrots are done, add that mixture over the quinoa. Sprinkle on the green onions and sesame seeds before serving.

Grab and Go Wraps

Ingredients:

- Julienned carrot (1)
- Red bell pepper (.5)
- Collard greens (4)
- Salt (.25 tsp.)
- Diced jalapeno pepper (.5)
- Diced shallot (1)
- Chopped cilantro leaves (.25 c.)
- Juiced lime (1)
- Avocado (1)
- Steamed green peas (1 c.)

Directions:

1. Take out your blender or your food processor and combine together the salt, jalapeno, shallot, cilantro, lime, avocado, and peas. The process to combine, but allow for a bit of texture to still be there.
2. Lay out the collard greens on the counter and then spread out your pea and avocado mixture to the top.
3. Add in the strips of carrots and bell peppers before rolling the collard greens up and securing with a toothpick.
4. Repeat with all of the Ingredients: before serving.

Nutty Tacos

Ingredients:

- Chopped cilantro (1 Tbsp.)
- Nutritional yeast (2 Tbsp.)
- Lettuce leaves, romaine (6)
- Cooked red quinoa (.25 c.)
- Salt (.25 tsp.)
- Tamari (1 tsp.)
- Coconut aminos (1 tsp.)
- Smoked paprika (.25 tsp.)
- Onion powder (.25 tsp.)
- Garlic powder (.25 tsp.)
- Chili powder (.25 tsp.)
- Ground coriander (1 tsp.)
- Ground cumin (1 tsp.)
- Olive oil (2 Tbsp.)
- Chopped sun-dried tomatoes (.25 c.)
- Slivered raw almonds (.25 c.)
- Walnuts (.5 c.)

Directions:

1. To begin with this recipe, add the almonds and walnuts in the food processor and pulse together until chopped.
2. Add in the tomatoes and pulse together a few times until you get a nice crumbly mixture.
3. From here, add in the salt, tamari, coconut aminos, paprika, onion, garlic, chili, coriander, cumin, and olive oil. Pulse a few more times to get fully combined.
4. Add the tomato and nut mixture into a bowl and combine together with the quinoa.
5. Divide this mixture between the leaves of romaine lettuce and top with the cilantro and nutritional yeast before serving.

Tex-Mex Bowl

Ingredients:

- Nutritional yeast (2 Tbsp.)
- Cilantro (2 Tbsp.)
- Sliced avocado (1)
- Salt (.25 tsp.)
- Olive oil (.25 c.)
- Apple cider vinegar (.25 c.)
- Juiced and zested lime (1)
- Juiced and zest lemon (1)
- Juiced oranges (2)
- Minced garlic cloves (2)
- Sliced red onion (1)
- Sliced bell peppers
- For the brown rice
- Back beans (.5 c.)
- Garlic powder (.5 tsp.)
- Cayenne pepper (.5 tsp.)
- Paprika (1 tsp.)
- Salt (1 tsp.)
- Garlic powder (1.5 tsp.)
- Chili powder (2 tsp.)
- Cooked brown rice (1 c.)
- Salsa
- Juice from one lime
- Salt (.25 tsp.)
- Diced cilantro (.25 c.)
- Diced red onion (.5)
- Diced tomatoes (2)

Directions:

1. Take out a big bowl and combine together the salt, olive oil, vinegar, lime zest and juice, lemon zest and juice, garlic, red onion, and the bell pepper.
2. Cover and let this set for about five hours to marinate a bit. While the peppers marinate a bit in the fridge, it is time to work on the salsa.
3. To make the salsa, add all of the Ingredients: in a small bowl and stir well to combine. Cover up the bowl and then place in the fridge.
4. In a medium bowl, add in all of the Ingredients: for the brown rice. Toss these together well and set to the side.
5. Heat up your skillet and add in the bell peppers with a bit of the marinade. Cook for a bit until the onion and bell peppers are soft.
6. Add the rice to some serving bowls and top with the bell peppers and onion mixture, the salsa, and the avocado. Top with the nutritional yeast and cilantro before serving.

Avocado Soup and Salmon

Ingredients:

- Cilantro (2 Tbsp.)
- Crushed pepper (1 tsp.)
- Olive oil (1 tsp.)
- Flaked salmon (1 can)
- Salt (.25 tsp.)
- Cumin (.25 tsp.)
- Vegetable broth (1.5 c.)
- Full fat coconut cream (2 Tbsp.)
- Lemon juice (4 Tbsp.)
- Sliced green onion (1 Tbsp.)
- Chopped shallot (1)
- Pitted avocados (3)

Directions:

1. Bring out a blender and combine together the salt, cumin, vegetable broth, coconut cream, two tablespoons of lemon juice, green onion, shallot, and avocado.
2. Blend this together until smooth and then chill in the fridge for an hour.
3. In the meantime, bring out a bowl and combine a tablespoon of the cilantro, two tablespoons of lemon juice, the pepper, olive oil, and salmon together.
4. Add the chilled avocado soup in the bowls and top each with the salmon along with the rest of the cilantro. Serve right away.

Asian Pumpkin Salad

Ingredients:

- Diced avocado (.5)
- Pomegranate seeds (.25 c.)
- Lemon juice (1 Tbsp.)
- Sliced kale (4 c.)
- Olive oil (1.5 Tbsp.)
- Cubed pumpkin (2 c.)
- Salt (.5 tsp.)
- Red chili flakes (.25 tsp.)
- Ground mustard (.25 tsp.)
- Ground garlic (.25 tsp.)
- Ground cloves (.25 tsp.)
- Black sesame seeds (1 Tbsp.)
- White sesame seeds (1 Tbsp.)

Directions:

1. Turn on the oven and give it time to heat up to 400 degrees. Prepare a baking tray with some parchment paper.
2. Using a large plate, combine both the black and white sesame seeds with the salt, chili flakes, mustard, garlic, and cloves.
3. Drizzle the pumpkin with a bit of olive oil and then roll each cube into the sesame seed mixture, pressing down a bit to coat.

4. Add the pumpkin to the baking tray and place into the oven. It will take half an hour to cook.
5. While the pumpkin is cooking, add the kale to a big bowl and drizzle on the salt, lemon juice, and the rest of the olive oil. Massage the mixture into the kale and then set aside.
6. When the pumpkin is done, add it on top of the kale and garnish with the avocado and pomegranate seeds before serving.

Sweet Potato Wraps

Ingredients:

- Avocado (1)
- Alfalfa sprouts (1 c.)
- Sliced red onion (.5)
- Spinach (1 c.)
- Cooked quinoa (.5 c.)
- Collard greens (4)
- Sweet potato hummus
- Crushed black pepper (.25 tsp.)
- Salt (.25 tsp.)
- Cinnamon powder (.25 tsp.)
- Chili powder (.25 tsp.)
- Garlic clove (1)
- Juiced lemon (.5)
- Olive oil (.25 c.)
- Tahini (.33 c.)
- Cubed sweet potato (1)

Directions:

1. Take the sweet potatoes and add them to a pan. Cover with the water and bring to a boil. When it reaches a boil, reduce the heat and let it cook for a bit to make the potatoes tender.
2. When these are done, drain out the water and add to the food processor along with the pepper, salt, cinnamon, chili powder, garlic, lemon juice, olive oil, and tahini. Process until smooth.
3. Lay out each of the collard greens and then spread the sweet potato hummus on each one.
4. Top this with the avocado, sprouts, onion, spinach, and quinoa. Roll these up and secure with toothpicks. Repeat until the greens and filling are gone.

Spicy Cabbage Bowl

Ingredients:

- Sesame seeds (1 Tbsp.)
- Green onion (.25 c.)
- Kale (2 c.)
- Coconut aminos (1 tsp.)
- Tamari (2 tsp.)
- Chopped cabbage kimchi (1 c.)
- Cooked brown rice (1 c.)
- Minced garlic (1 tsp.)
- Grated ginger (.5 tsp.)
- Sesame oil (2 tsp.)

Directions:

1. Bring out a skillet and heat up the sesame oil inside. When the oil is hot, add in the coconut aminos, tamari, kimchi, brown rice, garlic, and ginger together.
2. After five minutes of these Ingredients: cooking together, add in the green onions and kale and toss to combine.
3. Cook for a bit longer. Then you can garnish the dish with some sesame seeds before serving.

Citrus and Fennel Salad

Ingredients:

- Diced avocado (.5)
- Pomegranate seeds (2 Tbsp.)
- Pepper (.5 tsp.)
- Salt (.25 tsp.)
- Olive oil (.25 c.)
- Orange juice (2 Tbsp.)
- Lemon juice (2 Tbsp.)
- Chopped mint (1 Tbsp.)
- Chopped parsley (.5 c.)
- Sliced fennel bulbs (2)
- Segmented red grapefruit (.5)
- Segmented orange (1)

Directions:

1. To start this recipe, bring out a big bowl and combine together the parsley, mint, fennel slices, grapefruit segments, and orange segments. Toss to combine.
2. In another bowl, whisk together the pepper, salt, olive oil, orange juice, and lemon juice.
3. When that is combined, pour it over the fennel and citrus mixture in the big bowl, tossing around to coat.
4. Move the whole thing over to a plate and garnish with the avocado and the pomegranate seeds. Serve right away.

Vegan Burger

Servings: 4 Burger Patties

Ingredients:

- 1/4 to 1/2 cup spring water
- 1/2 teaspoon cayenne powder
- 1/2 teaspoon ginger powder
- Grapeseed oil
- 1 teaspoon dill
- 2 teaspoons sea salt
- 2 teaspoons onion powder
- 2 teaspoons oregano
- 2 teaspoons basil
- ¼ cup cherry tomatoes, diced
- 1/2 cup kale, diced
- 1/2 cup green peppers, diced
- 1/2 cup onions, diced
- 1 cup garbanzo bean flour

Directions:

1. Mix the vegetables and seasonings in a large bowl, then add in the flour. Gently add in spring water and stir the mixture until you have dough. In case the dough appears too loose, add in extra flour.
2. Divide the dough into 4 patties. Cook the patties in grapeseed oil, in a skillet over medium heat for approximately 2 to 3 minutes per side. Keep flipping until the burger is brown on all sides.
3. Serve the burger on a flatbread and enjoy.
4. Nutritional information per (2 burger patty) serving Calories: 413Carbs: 70.9g Protein: 21.8g Fat: 6g

---

Alkaline Spicy Kale

Servings: 1 serving

Ingredients:

- Grapeseed oil
- 1/4 teaspoon sea salt
- 1 teaspoon crushed red pepper
- 1/4 cup red pepper, diced
- 1/4 cup onion, diced
- 1 bunch of kale

Directions:

1. First wash the kale well, and then fold each kale leaf in half. Cut and discard the stems. Chop the prepared kale into bite-sized portions and use the salad spinner to remove water.

2. Into a wok, add in 2 tablespoons of grapeseed oil and heat the oil on high heat. Sauté the peppers and onions in oil for around 2-3 minutes and then season with some sea salt.
3. Lower the heat and add in kale, cover the wok with a lid and simmer for approximately 5 minutes.
4. Open the lid and add in crushed pepper, mix well and cover again. Cook until tender, or for about 3 additional minutes.
5. Nutritional information per (6 oz.) serving Calories: 52 Carbs: 10.8g Protein: 3g Fat: 0.7g

Electric Salad

Servings: 4

Ingredients:

- 3 jalapenos
- 2 red onions
- 1 orange pepper
- 1 yellow pepper
- 1 cup cherry tomatoes, chopped
- 1 bunch kale
- 1 handful romaine lettuce
- Extra virgin olive oil
- Juice of 1 lime

Directions:

1. First wash and rinse the Ingredients: well. Dry the Ingredients: and then cut them into bite-size pieces, or as required.
2. Put the Ingredients: in a bowl and drizzle with olive oil and the lime juice to your preferred taste.
3. Nutritional information per (7 oz.) serving: Calories: 85 Carbs: 34.8g Protein: 3g Fat: 0.5g

Kale Salad

Servings: 2

Ingredients:

- 1/4 teaspoon cayenne
- 1/2 teaspoon sea salt
- 1/2 cup cooked chickpeas
- 1/2 cup red onions
- 1/2 cup each of red, orange, yellow and green sliced bell peppers
- 4 cups chopped kale
- 1/2 cup Alkaline "Garlic" Sauce (recipe included).

- Alkaline Electric "Garlic" Sauce

Servings: 1 cup

Ingredients:

- 1/4 teaspoon dill
- 1/4 teaspoon sea salt
- 1/2 teaspoon ginger
- 1 tablespoon onion powder
- 1/4 cup shallots, minced
- 1 cup grapeseed oil

Directions:

1. In a bowl, mix all the Ingredients: for the kale salad and toss to mix.
2. Prepare the dressing by mixing together the Ingredients: for "Alkaline Electric Garlic Sauce".
3. Drizzle with half a cup of sauce and then serve.
4. Nutritional information per (7 oz.) serving: Calories: 183 Carbs: 28.3g Protein: 7.8g Fat: 5.1g

---

Walnuts, Dates, Orange and Kale Salad

Servings: 2

Ingredients:

- 1/2 red onion, very thinly sliced
- 2 bunches kale, or 6 packed cups of baby kale
- 6 medjool dates, pitted
- 1/3 cup whole walnuts
- For the dressing
- 5 tablespoons olive oil
- Pinch of coarse salt
- 1 medjool date
- 4 tablespoons orange juice, freshly squeezed
- 2 tablespoons lime juice

Directions:

1. Preheat the oven to 375 degrees F and then put walnuts on a baking dish. Roast the nuts for about 7-8 minutes, or until the skin begins to darken and split.
2. Once done, transfer the nuts while still hot and let them steam for 15 minutes while wrapped in a kitchen towel.
3. Once cooled down, squeeze and twist around firmly to remove the skin, all this time still wrapped in the towel.
4. In a food processor, put the pitted dates along with the nuts and pulse them until fully mixed and finely chopped. Set it aside to top the salad.
5. Then wash, dry and chop the kales and then put it in a large bowl. Slice the onion thinly and add into the bowl.

6. Now prepare the dressing by combining the **Ingredients:** for "dressing" in the blender apart from the olive oil.
7. Puree the mixture to break down the dates and then drizzle with the oil in a steady stream to emulsify the dressing.
8. Finally, toss the kale and onion mixture along with the orange-nut dressing together.
9. Move in a platter bowl and sprinkle with the nut and dates mixture. Enjoy!
10. Nutritional information per (7 oz.) serving: Calories: 645 Fat: 42.47g Carbohydrates: 71.08g Protein: 4.2g

---

Tomatoes with Basil-snack

Servings: 1 Serving

Ingredients:

- ¼ teaspoon sea salt
- 2 tablespoons lemon juice
- 2 tablespoons olive oil
- ¼ cup basil, fresh
- 1 cup chopped tomatoes, cherry or Roma

Directions:

1. Begin by slicing the cherry tomatoes and place in a medium-sized bowl.
2. Then chop your basil finely and add in the tomato bowl.
3. Drizzle some olive oil and lemon juice on the tomatoes and basil.
4. Add in some sea salt to taste.
5. Serve.
6. Nutritional information per (3 oz.) serving: Calories: 125 Fat: 13.57g Carbohydrates: 1.46g Protein: 0.22g

---

Spelt Pasta, Zucchini & Eggplant

Servings: 4

Ingredients:

- 2 teaspoons of dried basil leaves
- 1 teaspoon oregano
- 2/3 cup vegetable broth
- 2/3 cup sun dried cherry tomatoes, diced
- 1 large zucchini, diced
- 3 middle sized ripe cherry tomatoes, diced
- 2-3 ginger, crushed
- 1-2 white onions, finely diced
- 3 tablespoons extra virgin olive oil, cold pressed
- 1 large eggplant diced

- 300g spelt pasta
- Sea salt to taste

Directions:

1. Over medium heat, heat some oil in a pan and then stir-fry the eggplant, ginger and onion for about 8-10 minutes; while stirring persistently.
2. Then add the oregano, tomatoes and zucchini and let cook for 6-8 minutes, while stirring now and again.
3. Now heat up water and cook the pasta until firm to bite, and then add vegetable broth to the pan.
4. Season with fresh pepper, salt and dried basil. Allow the mixture to simmer for a few minutes, covered.
5. Once cooked through, you can serve the pasta sauce over the pasta and garnish with fresh basil leaves.
6. Nutritional information per (12 oz.) serving: Calories: 738 Fat: 49g Carbohydrates: 70.8g Protein: 14g

---

Alkalizing Millet Dish

Servings: 2

Ingredients:

- 1/2 teaspoon sea salt
- 2 1/2 cups water
- 1 cup millet

Directions:

1. Into a pot that has a closely-fitting lid, add in millet and then dry sauté on medium heat, stirring continuously.
2. As soon as the millet turns golden brown, add in the sea salt and water and cover the Ingredients: with a lid.
3. Then bring the mixture to a boil and let it simmer until all the water has been absorbed, or for about 25-35 minutes.
4. Alternatively, you can cook on an electric stove. Just cover the lid and bring to a boil, simmer for a couple of minutes and then turn off the cooker.
5. Leave the contents to cool for around 30 minutes with the lid still on to allow the millet to dry up.
6. Then serve and enjoy the millet.
7. Nutritional information per (14 oz.) serving: Calories: 378 Fat: 4.22g Carbohydrates: 72.85g Protein: 11.02g

Green Noodle Salad

Servings: 2

Ingredients:

- 1 pinch of sea salt
- 1 cup chopped fresh basil
- 2 tablespoons lemon juice, fresh
- ¼ cup yeast-free vegetable stock
- 1" ginger knob
- 1 cup kale
- 1 cup zucchini, chopped
- 1 handful lettuce
- 1 cup millet noodles

Directions:

1. First, cook the noodles based on the package Directions:. Once ready, drain and rinse using cold running water. Once done, set aside and allow to cool.
2. Cut the zucchini into thin slices and chop the kale. Steam the two vegetables very lightly for a few minutes until the color pops. Ensure they are still remain crunchy.
3. Wash and cut the lettuce and discard the stems.
4. Start preparing the dressing: combine vegetable stock and lemon juice in a grinder, and then add in chopped ginger. Mix the Ingredients: for approximately 15-30 seconds.
5. Now mix the basil, chopped lettuce, zucchini, kale and noodles in a bowl and pour over the dressing. Combine well and then season with salt.
6. Serve and enjoy.
7. Nutritional information per (9 oz.) serving: Calories: 303 Fat: 3.28g Carbohydrates: 52g Protein: 18.7g

---

Squash Ratatouille

Servings: 4

Ingredients:

- 1 cup spring water
- Pinch of cayenne pepper
- Sea salt or organic salt
- 4 tablespoons extra-virgin olive oil, cold pressed
- 2 teaspoons thyme
- 1 fennel bulb
- 2 big onions
- 1 cup cherry tomatoes, chopped
- 1 red bell pepper
- 1 yellow bell pepper
- 16 ounces fresh squash

Directions:

1. Cut the bell pepper, tomatoes and the squash fresh into bit-sized portions. Then dice fennel and the onions.
2. In a pot, heat some olive oil and then sauté the fennel and onions for a few minutes.
3. Now add in the bell pepper and squash. Then stir-fry the mixture for approximately 8 minutes or so.
4. Once done, add the alkaline water, thyme and tomatoes and now cook until the veggies are quite tender yet not too soft.
5. Nutritional information per (14 oz.) serving: Calories: 263 Fat: 14.17g Carbohydrates: 35.39g Protein: 3.78g

Roasted Vegetables

Servings: 2

Ingredients:

- A drizzle of cayenne pepper
- A drizzle of olive oil
- 2 fennel bulbs, chopped
- 1/2 onion, sliced
- 1 yellow squash, sliced
- 1 zucchini, sliced
- 1 bunch of green beans, ends cut off

Directions:

1. Preheat your oven to 450 degrees F.
2. Then on a lipped baking sheet, put the fennel bulbs and vegetables and then drizzle some olive oil all over.
3. Add some cayenne pepper and stir.
4. Bake the vegetables for about 16 minutes, while stirring at 8 minutes interval.
5. Soon as the veggies are slightly browned, remove from heat and serve.
6. Nutritional information per (10 oz.) serving: Calories: 70 Fat: 1.87g Carbohydrates: 13.23g Protein: 2.39g

Crockpot Summer Veggies

Servings: 6

Ingredients:

- 1 tablespoon chopped thyme, fresh
- 2 tablespoons chopped basil, fresh
- ½ cup olive oil
- Juice of 1 lemon

- 1 cup sliced mushrooms
- 2 ½ cups sliced zucchini
- 2 cups sliced bell pepper, yellow
- 1 ½ cups chopped onions
- 1 cup chopped cherry tomatoes
- 2 cups slice okra

Directions:

1. Mix the veggies in a bowl, then mix olive oil and lemon juice in a separate bowl.
2. Stir in thyme and basil and put the veggies in a slow cooker. Top with marinade and stir to coat.
3. Cook the veggies on high heat for 3 hours, while stirring every hour.
4. Once cooked through, serve and enjoy.
5. Nutritional information per (9 oz.) serving: Calories: 313 Fat: 27.21g Carbohydrates: 18.53g Protein: 2.6g

---

Brazilian Kale

Servings: 2

Ingredients:

- Juice of 1/2 lime
- 1/4 teaspoon cayenne pepper
- 1/4 teaspoon salt
- 2 bunches kale, thin strips
- 2 fennel bulbs, peeled, chopped and smashed
- 2 tablespoons olive oil

Directions:

1. Remove the stocks, from the kale, stack the leaf halves together and slice the kale.
2. Smash the fennel bulbs using the flat end of chef's knife or a pestle and mortar.
3. In a large skillet, heat olive oil on medium for a minute and then add in fennel.
4. Sauté for 1 minute or until it becomes aromatic, and then add in cayenne pepper, salt and kale.
5. Lower the heat to medium low and sauté to soften the greens and achieve vibrant color or for approximately 3-4 minutes.
6. Then squeeze the lime juice and add in more salt and cayenne pepper if required. Serve and enjoy.
7. Nutritional information per (12 oz.) serving: Calories: 228 Fat: 14g Carbohydrates: 24.01g Protein: 5.8g

Instant Pot Zucchini and Tomato Mélange

Servings: 4

Ingredients:

- 1 bunch of basil
- Swirls of fresh olive oil
- 1 fennel bulb, chopped nicely
- 1 teaspoon salt
- 1 cup cherry tomato puree
- 2 cups chopped cherry tomatoes
- 6 medium zucchini, roughly chopped
- 1 tablespoon olive oil
- 2 medium onions, roughly chopped

Directions:

1. Pre-heat your Instant Pot as you slice the onion. Add oil and onion and cook for 5 minutes. Chop the zucchini.
2. Once the onion becomes translucent, add in zucchini, cherry tomatoes, puree and pinch of salt.
3. Lock the lid and cook for 5 minutes at high pressure. Then quick release pressure and mix in the fennel.
4. Using a slotted spoon, strain out the veggies and serve with fresh basil leaves and olive oil.
5. Refrigerate the cooking liquid for use as chilled soup of base stock to make risotto.
6. Nutritional information per (12 oz.) serving: Calories: 130 Fat: 7.3g Carbohydrates: 15.62g Protein: 3.27g

Seaweed Wraps with Quinoa and Veggies

Servings: 2 Wraps

Ingredients:

- 1 tablespoon sesame seed oil
- 1 tablespoon raw sesame seeds
- 1 teaspoon fresh ginger root, finely grated
- 1 teaspoon seeded and finely chopped fresh red chili
- 1 finely chopped fennel bulb
- ¼ cup finely chopped fresh culantro leaves
- ¼ cup raw cucumber sticks
- ¼ cup raw parsnips
- ½ cup cooked quinoa

Directions:

1. Spread 2 nori sheets individually on a working surface.

2. Mix the quinoa with chili, ginger, fennel, seeds and culantro leaves.
3. Into this mixture, add in sesame seed oil and blend well.
4. Distribute the seed mix and quinoa mixture between two nori sheets, putting it along the edge of each sheet.
5. Top the quinoa mixture with parsnip sticks and cucumber. Now roll the sheets and gently wrap the contents in them.
6. You may slide up the nori rolls to appear like sushi rolls, if you like.
7. Nutritional information per (8 oz.) serving: Calories: 159 Fat: 7.35g Carbohydrates: 23g Protein: 5.6g

---

Lettuce Wraps

Servings: 4 Wraps

Ingredients:

- ½ cup roughly chopped raw walnuts
- ½ cup fresh strawberries, sliced
- ½ of a ripe avocado, pitted and sliced
- 1 cup raw green beans
- 4 large lettuce leaves

Directions:

1. Spread out the lettuce leaves on a kitchen work surface or a plate.
2. Share the green beans between individual lettuce leaves, putting them at a 90 degree angle to the edge.
3. Now share the avocado slices between individual lettuce leaves putting them on top of the spears.
4. Also share the berries between individual lettuce leaves and put them on top of the avocado.
5. Then share the nuts between the lettuce leaves and put them on top of the berries.
6. Finally roll up the leaves, and wrap all the contents in them.
7. Nutritional information per Wrap: Calories: 225 Fat: 11.5g Carbohydrates: 28g Protein: 9g

Rainbow Salad with Meyer Lemon Dressing

Servings: 4

Ingredients:

- 1/2 avocado, sliced
- Micro green or sprouts
- 1 cup pea shoots
- ½ yellow pepper, sliced
- 1/8 red onion, thinly sliced
- ½ cup diced cherry tomatoes
- 1 parsnip, ribbon with peeler
- Arugula and other greens
- Raw walnuts chopped or slivered
- For the Dressing

- 1 tablespoon agave sugar
- 1/16 teaspoon of sea salt
- 1/6 cup of cold pressed extra virgin olive oil
- 3 stems of fresh dill
- 3 basil leaves
- 3/4 teaspoon of chopped red onion
- ½ avocado
- 1 Meyer lemon, juiced

Directions:

1. Put a handful of arugula in each of the serving bowls.
2. Add the rest of the vegetables followed by micro greens and the pea shoots.
3. Then top with the nuts and set aside.
4. Now move the Ingredients: for the dressing in a blender and puree until smooth and creamy.
5. Pour the dressing into a serving bowl and then drizzle it over the salad and enjoy!
6. Nutritional information per (8 oz.) serving: Calories: 422 Fat: 35.8g Carbohydrates: 24.45g Protein: 6g

---

Alkaline Quinoa & Hummus Wraps

Servings: 4 Wraps

Ingredients:

- 1 cup avocado
- 1 cup hummus
- 1 cup quinoa
- 1/2 cup parsnips

- 1/2 cup lettuce
- 1/2 cup sprouts
- 4 large baby kale

Directions:

1. Place a cup of quinoa in a pan along with 2 cups of water. Bring the water to a boil and lower the heat to simmer until the quinoa is fluffy and water has evaporated.
2. Cut the kale leaves off the plant, wash them and lay them as a regular wrap. Layer the hummus on each of the kale to help hold other Ingredients: in place.

3. Now slice and place the avocado in a line right from the top to bottom and down the middle of the kale leaf.
4. Once done, put the quinoa equally between the kale leaves and fill up with the rest of the Ingredients:.
5. Finally wrap the leaf. Just fold at the bottom and now roll it up. Consider using a toothpick to help hold things in place.
6. Nutritional information per wrap: Calories: 352 Fat: 13.61g Carbohydrates: 48.43g Protein: 11.2g

Grilled Courgettes Salad

Servings: 2

Ingredients:

- 3 oz. watercress
- 6 courgettes
- Sea salt
- Chilli-Mint Dressing:
- 6 tablespoons extra virgin olive oil
- ½ cup fresh basil leaves
- 1 red chili
- Zest and juice of 1/2 a lemon
- Cayenne pepper
- Salt

Directions:

1. Clean the watercress and the courgettes. Then slice the courgettes into thin strips. Season the strips with salt and let them soften slightly in salt.
2. Meanwhile, begin to prepare the dressing. Just wash the basil leaves, chili and lemon and set aside.
3. Discard seeds from the chili and chop it well. Then shred the leaves and set aside.
4. In a bowl, whisk together olive oil, basil, chili and lemon zest and then season with cayenne pepper and salt. Now put watercress in a serving platter.
5. Fire up your barbecue for direct heat at 220 degrees F. Put the salt-softened strips on a grate and lock the lid in place.
6. Now grill the courgettes until grill marks develop, or for approximately 3 to 4 minutes per side.
7. Then remove them from the grill and let them cool down. To serve, put the courgettes on the watercress then drizzle the dressing on top.
8. Nutritional information per (6 oz.) serving: Calories: 177 Fat: 18.2g Carbohydrates: 2.25g Protein: 2.85g

Creamy Kale Salad With Avocado And Tomato

Servings: 2

Ingredients:

- 1/2 teaspoon of cayenne pepper
- 1 tablespoons agave syrup
- 1 funnel bulb, chopped
- Juice of 1 lime
- ½ cup chopped cherry tomatoes
- 1 ripe medium avocado
- 2 large handfuls kale

Directions:

1. Clean and chop tomatoes and kales and then put them in a mixing bowl or large glass bowl.
2. Then peel the avocado and put it into the mixing bowl.
3. Juice the lime and now add it along with the rest of the Ingredients: to the mixing bowl.
4. Rub the Ingredients: together then serve the salad.
5. Nutritional information per (11 oz.) serving: Calories: 285 Fat: 15.94g Carbohydrates: 36.57g Protein: 7.56g

---

Sesame Ginger Rice

Servings: 4

Ingredients:

- 1/2 teaspoon Celtic sea salt
- 2 teaspoons fresh lime juice
- ½ cup culantro, finely chopped
- 4 cups mushrooms (any type except shiitake), finely chopped
- 6 green onions, finely chopped
- 1 fennel bulb, chopped
- 2 tablespoons minced fresh ginger
- 1 small green chile, ribbed, seeded, and minced
- 2 tablespoons toasted sesame oil
- 2 tablespoons grapeseed oil
- 1 cup wild cooked rice

Directions:

1. Heat oil in a deep skillet or wok over medium high heat.
2. Once hot, sauté mushrooms, green onions, fennel, ginger and chile along with some salt until soft and combined, or for approximately 5 minutes.
3. Add in tamari and rice and keep on heat for additional 2-3 minutes.
4. Add in lime juice, culantro and ¼ teaspoon salt and enjoy.
5. Nutritional information per (12 oz.) serving: Calories: 340 Fat: 12.06g Carbohydrates: 46.45g Protein: 16g

Chapter 6. Dinner

Vegetable Soup

Preparation time: 15 minutes

Cooking time: 25 minutes.

Servings: 3

Ingredients:

- ½ tbsp olive oil
- 2 tbsp onion, chopped
- 2 tsp garlic, minced
- ½ cup carrots, peeled and chopped
- ½ cup green cabbage, chopped
- 1/3 cup French beans, chopped
- 3 cups homemade vegetable broth
- ½ tbsp fresh lemon juice
- 3 tbsp water
- 2 tbsp arrowroot starch
- Sea salt and freshly ground black pepper, to taste

Directions:

1. Heat the oil in a large, heavy bottomed pan over medium heat and sauté the onion and garlic for about 4-5 minutes.
2. Add the carrots, cabbage, and beans and cook for about 4-5 minutes, stirring frequently.
3. Stir in the broth and bring to a boil.
4. Cook for about 4-5 minutes.
5. Meanwhile, in a small bowl, dissolve the arrowroot starch in water.
6. Slowly, add the arrowroot starch mixture, stirring continuously.
7. Cook for about 7-8 minutes, stirring occasionally.
8. Stir in the lemon juice, salt, and black pepper and remove from the heat.
9. Serve hot.

Nutrition: Calories 163; Total Fat 4.2 g; Saturated Fat 0.8 g; Cholesterol 0 mg; Sodium 861 mg; Total Carbs 22.5 g; Fiber 6.3 g; Sugar 2.3 g; Protein 9.2 g

---

Lentil & Spinach Soup

Preparation time: 15 minutes

Cooking time: 1¼ hours. Total time: 1½ hours

Servings: 6

Ingredients:

- 2 tbsp olive oil
- 2 carrots, peeled and chopped

- 2 celery stalks, chopped
- 2 sweet onions, chopped
- 3 garlic cloves, minced
- 1½ cups brown lentils, rinsed
- 2 cups tomatoes, chopped finely
- ¼ tsp dried basil, crushed
- ¼ tsp dried oregano, crushed
- ¼ tsp dried thyme, crushed
- 1 tsp ground cumin
- ½ tsp ground coriander
- ½ tsp paprika
- 6 cups vegetable broth
- 3 cups fresh spinach, chopped
- Sea salt and freshly ground black pepper, to taste
- 2 tbsp fresh lemon juice

Directions:

1. In a large soup pan, heat the oil over medium heat and sauté the carrot, celery, and onion for about 5 minutes.
2. Add the garlic and sauté for about 1 minute.
3. Add the lentils and sauté for about 3 minutes.
4. Stir in the tomatoes, herbs, spices, and broth and bring to a boil.
5. Reduce the heat to low and simmer partially covered for about 1 hour or until desired doneness
6. Stir in the spinach, salt, and black pepper and cook for about 4 minutes.
7. Stir in the lemon juice and remove from the heat.
8. Serve hot.

Nutrition: Calories 258; Total Fat 1.5 g; Saturated Fat 0.1 g; Cholesterol 0 mg; Sodium 90 mg; Total Carbs 63.6 g; Fiber 13.7 g; Sugar 45.4 g; Protein 5.3 g

---

Veggie Stew

Preparation time: 20 minutes

Cooking time: 35 minutes.

Servings: 8

Ingredients:

- 2 tbsp coconut oil
- 1 large sweet onion, chopped
- 1 medium parsnip, peeled and chopped
- 3 tbsp homemade tomato paste
- 2 large garlic cloves, minced
- ½ tsp ground cinnamon
- ½ tsp ground ginger
- 1 tsp ground cumin
- ¼ tsp cayenne pepper
- 2 medium carrots, peeled and chopped
- 2 medium purple potatoes, peeled and chopped
- 2 medium sweet potatoes, peeled and chopped
- 4 cups homemade vegetable broth

- 2 cups fresh kale, trimmed and chopped
- 2 tbsp fresh lemon juice
- Sea salt and freshly ground black pepper, to taste

Directions:

1. In a large soup pan, melt the coconut oil over medium-high heat and sauté the onion for about 5 minutes.
2. Add the parsnip and sauté for about 3 minutes.
3. Stir in the tomato paste, garlic, and spices and sauté for about 2 minutes.
4. Stir in carrots, potatoes, sweet potatoes, and broth and bring to a boil.
5. Reduce the heat to medium-low and simmer covered for about 20 minutes.
6. Stir in the kale, lemon juice, salt, and black pepper and simmer for about 5 minutes.
7. Serve hot.

Nutrition: Calories 258; Total Fat 1.5 g; Saturated Fat 0.1 g; Cholesterol 0 mg; Sodium 90 mg; Total Carbs 63.6 g; Fiber 13.7 g; Sugar 45.4 g; Protein 5.3 g

---

Quinoa & Lentil Stew

Preparation time: 15 minutes

Cooking time: 30 minutes.

Servings: 6

Ingredients:

- 1 tbsp coconut oil
- 3 carrots, peeled and chopped
- 3 celery stalks, chopped
- 1 yellow onion, chopped
- 4 garlic cloves, minced
- 4 cups tomatoes, chopped
- 1 cup red lentils, rinsed and drained
- ½ cup dried quinoa, rinsed and drained
- 1½ tsp ground cumin
- 1 tsp red chili powder
- 5 cups vegetable broth
- 2 cups fresh spinach, chopped
- Sea salt and freshly ground black pepper, to taste

Directions:

1. In a large pan, heat the oil over medium heat and sauté the celery, onion, and carrot for about 4-5 minutes.
2. Add the garlic and sauté for about 1 minute.
3. Add the remaining Ingredients: except the spinach and bring to a boil.
4. Reduce the heat to low and simmer covered for about 20 minutes.
5. Stir in spinach and simmer for about 3-4 minutes.
6. Stir in the salt and black pepper and remove from the heat.

7. Serve hot.

Nutrition: Calories 292; Total Fat 6.9 g; Saturated Fat 1.2 g; Cholesterol 0 mg; Sodium 842 mg; Total Carbs 39.1 g; Fiber 17.3 g; Sugar 6.1 g; Protein 19 g

---

Black Bean Chili

Preparation time: 15 minutes

Cooking time: 2 hours 10 minutes. Total time: 2 hours 25 minutes

Servings: 6

Ingredients:

- 2 tbsp olive oil
- 1 onion, chopped
- 1 small red bell pepper, seeded and chopped
- 1 small green bell pepper, seeded and chopped
- 4 garlic cloves, minced
- 1 tsp ground cumin
- 1 tsp cayenne pepper
- 1 tbsp red chili powder
- 1 medium sweet potato, peeled and chopped
- 3 cups tomatoes, chopped finely
- 4 cups cooked black beans, rinsed and drained
- 2 cups homemade vegetable broth
- Sea salt and freshly ground black pepper, to taste

Directions:

1. In a large pan, heat the oil over medium-high heat and sauté the onion and bell peppers for about 3-4 minutes.
2. Add the garlic and spices and sauté for about 1 minute.
3. Add the sweet potato and cook for about 4-5 minutes.
4. Add the remaining Ingredients: and bring to a boil.
5. Reduce the heat to medium-low and simmer covered for about 1½-2 hours.
6. Season with the salt and black pepper and remove from the heat.
7. Serve hot.

Nutrition: Calories 275; Total Fat 7.2 g; Saturated Fat 0.9 g; Cholesterol 0 mg; Sodium 613 mg; Total Carbs 40.8 g; Fiber 11.2 g; Sugar 12 g; Protein 13.1 g

Kidney Bean Curry

Preparation time: 15 minutes

Cooking time: 25 minutes.

Servings: 6

Ingredients:

- ¼ cup extra-virgin olive oil
- 1 medium onion, chopped finely
- 2 garlic cloves, minced
- 2 tbsp fresh ginger, minced
- 1 cup homemade tomato puree
- 1 tsp ground coriander
- 1 tsp ground cumin
- ½ tsp ground turmeric
- ¼ tsp cayenne pepper
- Sea salt and freshly ground black pepper, to taste
- 2 large plum tomatoes, chopped finely
- 3 cups boiled red kidney beans
- 2 cups water
- ½ cup fresh parsley, chopped

Directions:

1. In a large soup pan, heat the oil over medium heat and sauté the onion, garlic, and ginger for about 4-5 minutes.
2. Stir in the tomato puree and spices and cook for about 5 minutes.
3. Stir in the tomatoes, kidney beans, and water and bring to a boil over high heat.
4. Reduce the heat to medium and simmer for about 10-15 minutes or until desired thickness.
5. Serve hot and garnish with parsley.

Nutrition: Calories 228; Total Fat 9.9 g; Saturated Fat 1.3 g; Cholesterol 0 mg; Sodium 341 mg; Total Carbs 28.1 g; Fiber 8.4 g; Sugar 5.5 g; Protein 8.9 g

Green Bean Casserole

Preparation time: 20 minutes

Cooking time: 20 minutes.

Servings: 6

Ingredients:

- For Onion Slices:
- ½ cup yellow onion, sliced very thinly
- ¼ cup almond flour
- 1/8 tsp garlic powder

- Sea salt and freshly ground black pepper, to taste
- For Casserole:
- 1 lb fresh green beans, trimmed
- 1 tbsp olive oil
- 8 oz fresh cremini mushrooms, sliced
- ½ cup yellow onion, sliced thinly
- 1/8 tsp garlic powder
- Sea salt and freshly ground black pepper, to taste
- 1 tsp fresh thyme, chopped
- ½ cup homemade vegetable broth
- ½ cup coconut cream

Directions:

1. Preheat the oven to 350 degrees F.
2. For onion slices, place all the Ingredients: in a bowl and toss them to coat the onion well.
3. Arrange the onion slices onto a large baking sheet in a single layer and set it aside.
4. In a pan of salted boiling water, add the green beans and cook for about 5 minutes.
5. Drain the green beans and transfer them into a bowl of ice water.
6. Again, drain well and transfer them again into a large bowl. Set them aside.
7. In a large skillet, heat oil over medium-high heat and sauté the mushrooms, onion, garlic powder, salt, and black pepper for about 2-3 minutes.
8. Stir in the thyme and broth and cook for about 3-5 minutes or until all the liquid is absorbed.
9. Remove from the heat and transfer the mushroom mixture into the bowl with the green beans.
10. Add the coconut cream and stir to combine well.
11. Transfer the mixture into a 10-inch casserole dish.
12. Place the casserole dish and baking sheet of onion slices into the oven.
13. Bake for about 15-17 minutes.
14. Remove the baking dish and sheet from the oven and let it cool for about 5 minutes before serving.
15. Top the casserole with the crispy onion slices evenly.
16. Cut into 6 equal-sized portions and serve.

Nutrition: Calories 138; Total Fat 9.7 g; Saturated Fat 4.8 g; Cholesterol 0 mg; Sodium 101 mg; Total Carbs 11.1 g; Fiber 4.2 g; Sugar 3.4 g; Protein 4.4 g

Vegetarian Pie

Preparation time: 20 minutes

Cooking time: 1 hour 20 minutes

Servings: 8

Ingredients:

- For Topping:
- 5 cups water
- 1¼ cups yellow cornmeal
- For Filing:
- 1 tbsp extra-virgin olive oil
- 1 large onion, chopped
- 1 medium red bell pepper, seeded and chopped
- 2 garlic cloves, minced
- 1 tsp dried oregano, crushed
- 2 tsp chili powder
- 2 cups fresh tomatoes, chopped
- 2½ cups cooked pinto beans
- 2 cups boiled corn kernels

Directions:

1. Preheat the oven to 375 degrees F. Lightly grease a shallow baking dish.
2. In a pan, add the water over medium-high heat and bring to a boil.
3. Slowly, add the cornmeal, stirring continuously.
4. Reduce the heat to low and cook covered for about 20 minutes, stirring occasionally.
5. Meanwhile, prepare the filling. In a large skillet, heat the oil over medium heat and sauté the onion and bell pepper for about 3-4 minutes.
6. Add the garlic, oregano, and spices and sauté for about 1 minute
7. Add the remaining Ingredients: and stir to combine.
8. Reduce the heat to low and simmer for about 10-15 minutes, stirring occasionally.
9. Remove from the heat.
10. Place half of the cooked cornmeal into the prepared baking dish evenly.
11. Place the filling mixture over the cornmeal evenly.
12. Place the remaining cornmeal over the filling mixture evenly.
13. Bake for 45-50 minutes or until the top becomes golden brown.
14. Remove the pie from the oven and set it aside for about 5 minutes before serving.

Nutrition: Calories 350; Total Fat 3.9 g; Saturated Fat 0.6 g; Cholesterol 0 mg; Sodium 34 mg; Total Carbs 65 g; Fiber 13.3 g; Sugar 5.4 g; Protein 16.6 g

Rice & Lentil Loaf

Preparation time: 20 minutes

Cooking time: 1 hour 50 minutes. Total time: 2 hours 10 minutes

Servings: 8

Ingredients:

- 1¾ cups plus 2 tbsp filtered water, divided
- ½ cup wild rice
- ½ cup brown lentils
- Pinch of sea salt
- ½ tsp no-sodium Italian seasoning
- 1 medium yellow onion, chopped
- 1 celery stalk, chopped
- 6 cremini mushrooms, chopped
- 4 garlic cloves, minced
- ¾ cup rolled oats
- ½ cup pecans, chopped finely
- ¾ cup homemade tomato sauce
- ½ tsp red pepper flakes, crushed
- 1 tsp fresh rosemary, minced
- 2 tsp fresh thyme, minced

Directions:

1. In a pan, add 1¾ cups of water, rice, lentils, salt, and Italian seasoning and bring them to a boil over medium-high heat.
2. Reduce the heat to low and simmer covered for about 45 minutes.
3. Remove from the heat and set it aside still covered for at least 10 minutes.
4. Preheat the oven to 350 degrees F.
5. With parchment paper, line a 9x5-inch loaf pan.
6. In a skillet, heat the remaining water over medium heat and sauté the onion, celery, mushrooms, and garlic for about 4-5 minutes.
7. Remove from the heat and let it cool slightly.
8. In a large mixing bowl, add the oats, pecans, tomato sauce, and fresh herbs and mix until well combined.
9. Combine the rice mixture and vegetable mixture with the oat mixture and mix well.
10. In a blender, add the mixture and pulse until a chunky mixture forms.
11. Transfer the mixture into the prepared loaf pan evenly.
12. With a piece of foil, cover the loaf pan and bake it for about 40 minutes.
13. Uncover and bake for about 15-20 minutes more or until the top becomes golden brown.
14. Remove it from the oven and set it aside for about 5-10 minutes before slicing.
15. Cut into desired sized slices and serve.

Nutrition: Calories 179; Total Fat 6.6 g; Saturated Fat 0.7 g; Cholesterol 0 mg; Sodium 157 mg; Total Carbs 24.6 g; Fiber 6.8 g; Sugar 2.6 g; Protein 7.1 g

Asparagus Risotto

Preparation time: 15 minutes

Cooking time: 45 minutes. Total time: 1 hour

Servings: 4

Ingredients:

- 15-20 fresh asparagus spears, trimmed and cut into 1½-inch pieces
- 2 tbsp olive oil
- 1 cup yellow onion, chopped
- 1 garlic clove, minced
- 1 cup Arborio rice
- 1 tbsp fresh lemon zest, grated finely
- 2 tbsp fresh lemon juice
- 5½ cups hot vegetable broth
- 1 tbsp fresh parsley, chopped
- ¼ cup nutritional yeast
- Sea salt and freshly ground black pepper, to taste

Directions:

1. Boil water in a medium pan then add asparagus and cook for about 3 minutes.
2. Drain the asparagus and rinse under cold running water.
3. Drain well and set aside.
4. In a large pan heat oil over medium heat and sauté the onion for about 5 minutes.
5. Add the garlic and sauté for about 1 minute.
6. Add the rice and stir fry for about 2 minutes.
7. Add the lemon zest, lemon juice, and ½ cup of broth and cook for about 3 minutes or until all the liquid is absorbed, stirring gently.
8. Add 1 cup of broth and cook until all the broth is absorbed.
9. While stirring occasionally, repeat this process by adding ¾ cup of broth at a time until all the broth is absorbed. (This procedure will take about 20-30 minutes.)
10. Stir in the cooked asparagus and remaining Ingredients: and cook for about 4 minutes.
11. Serve hot.

Nutrition: Calories 353; Total Fat 9.9 g; Saturated Fat 1.8 g; Cholesterol 0 mg; Sodium 1,100 mg; Total Carbs 50.5 g; Fiber 6.5 g; Sugar 4.1 g; Protein 16.9 g

Quinoa & Chickpea Salad

Preparation time: 15 minutes

Cooking time: 45 minutes

Servings: 8

Ingredients:

- 1¾ cups homemade vegetable broth
- 1 cup quinoa, rinsed
- Sea salt, to taste
- 1½ cups cooked chickpeas
- 1 medium green bell pepper, seeded and chopped
- 1 medium red bell pepper, seeded and chopped
- 2 cucumbers, chopped
- ½ cup scallion (green part only), chopped
- 1 tablespoon olive oil
- 2 tablespoons fresh cilantro leaves, chopped

Directions:

1. In a pan, add the broth and bring to a boil over high heat.
2. Add the quinoa and salt and cook until boiling again.
3. Reduce the heat to low and simmer covered for about 15-20 minutes or until all the liquid is absorbed.
4. Remove from the heat and set aside still covered for about 5-10 minutes.
5. Uncover and fluff the quinoa with a fork.
6. In a large serving bowl, add the quinoa and the remaining Ingredients: and gently toss to coat.
7. Serve immediately.

Nutrition: Calories 348 Total Fat 7.7 g Saturated Fat 1 g Cholesterol 0 mg Sodium 280 mg Total Carbs 56 g Fiber 11.9 g Sugar 9.4 g Protein 16.3 g

Mixed Veggie Soup

Ingredients:

- 1½ tablespoons olive oil
- 4 medium carrots, peeled and chopped
- 1 medium onion, chopped
- 2 garlic cloves, minced
- 2 celery stalks, chopped
- 2 cups fresh tomatoes, chopped finely
- 3 cups small cauliflower florets
- 3 cups small broccoli florets
- 3 cups frozen peas
- 8 cups homemade vegetable broth
- 3 tablespoons fresh lemon juice

- Sea salt, to taste

Directions:

1. In a large soup pan, heat the oil over medium heat and sauté the carrots, celery, and onion for 6 minutes.
2. Stir in the garlic and sauté for about 1 minute.
3. Add the tomatoes and cook for about 2-3 minutes, crushing them with the back of a spoon.
4. Add the vegetables and broth and bring to a boil over high heat.
5. Reduce the heat to low.
6. Cover the pan and simmer for about 30-35 minutes.
7. Mix in the lemon juice and salt and remove from the heat.
8. Serve hot.

Nutrition: Calories 1587 Total Fat 4.5 g Saturated Fat 0.9 g Cholesterol 0 mg Sodium 888 mg Total Carbs 20.1 g Fiber 6.9 g Sugar 8.4 g Protein 10.5 g

---

Beans & Barley Soup

Preparation time: 15 minutes

Cooking time: 40 minutes

Servings: 4

Ingredients:

- 1 tablespoon olive oil
- 1 white onion, chopped
- 2 celery stalks, chopped
- 1 large carrot, peeled and chopped
- 2 tablespoons fresh rosemary, chopped
- 2 garlic cloves, minced
- 4 cups fresh tomatoes, chopped
- 4 cups homemade vegetable broth
- 1 cup pearl barley
- 2 cups cooked white beans
- 2 tablespoons fresh lemon juice
- 4 tablespoons fresh parsley leaves, chopped

Directions:

1. In a large soup pan, heat the oil over medium heat and sauté the onion, celery, and carrot for about 4-5 minutes.
2. Add the garlic and rosemary and sauté for about 1 minute.
3. Add the tomatoes and cook for 3-4 minutes, crushing them with the back of a spoon.
4. Add the barley and broth and bring to a boil.
5. Reduce the heat to low and simmer covered for about 20-25 minutes.

6. Stir in the beans and lemon juice and simmer for about 5 minutes more.
7. Garnish with parsley and serve hot

Nutrition: Calories 407 Total Fat 7.2 g Saturated Fat 1.2 g Cholesterol 0 mg Sodium 841 mg Total Carbs 70.3 g Fiber 16.9 g Sugar 8.2 g Protein 18.3 g

---

Tofu & Bell Pepper Stew

Preparation time: 15 minutes

Cooking time: 15 minutes

Servings: 6

Ingredients:

- 2 tablespoons garlic
- 1 jalapeño pepper, seeded and chopped
- 1 (16-ounce) jar roasted red peppers, rinsed, drained, and chopped
- 2 cups homemade vegetable broth
- 2 cups filtered water
- 1 medium green bell pepper, seeded and sliced thinly
- 1 medium red bell pepper, seeded and sliced thinly
- 1 (16-ounce) package extra-firm tofu, drained and cubed
- 1 (10-ounce) package frozen baby spinach, thawed

Directions:

1. Add the garlic, jalapeño pepper, and roasted red peppers in a food processor and pulse until smooth.
2. In a large pan, add the puree, broth, and water and cook until boiling over medium-high heat.
3. Add the bell peppers and tofu and stir to combine.
4. Reduce the heat to medium and cook for about 5 minutes.
5. Stir in the spinach and cook for about 5 minutes.
6. Serve hot.

Nutrition: Calories 130 Total Fat 5.3 g Saturated Fat 0.6 g Cholesterol 0 mg Sodium 482 mg Total Carbs 12.2 g Fiber 2.9 g Sugar 6.2 g Protein 11.8 g

Chickpea Stew

Preparation time: 15 minutes

Cooking time: 30 minutes

Servings: 4

Ingredients:

- 1 tablespoon olive oil
- 1 medium onion, chopped
- 2 cups carrots, peeled and chopped
- 2 garlic cloves, minced
- 1 teaspoon red pepper flakes
- 2 large tomatoes, peeled, seeded, and chopped finely
- 2 cups homemade vegetable broth
- 2 cups cooked chickpeas
- 2 cups fresh spinach, chopped
- 1 tablespoon fresh lemon juice
- Sea salt and freshly ground black pepper, to taste

Directions:

1. In a large pan, heat oil over medium heat and sauté the onion and carrot for about 6 minutes.
2. Stir in the garlic and red pepper flakes and sauté for about 1 minute.
3. Add the tomatoes and cook for about 2-3 minutes.
4. Add the broth and bring to a boil.
5. Reduce the heat to low and simmer for about 10 minutes.
6. Stir in the chickpeas and simmer for about 5 minutes.
7. Stir in the spinach and simmer for 3-4 minutes more.
8. Stir in the lemon juice and seasoning and remove from the heat.
9. Serve hot.

Nutrition: Calories 217 Total Fat 6.6 g Saturated Fat 0.8 g Cholesterol 0 mg Sodium 827 mg Total Carbs 31.4 g Fiber 9.5 g Sugar 7.8 g Protein 10.6 g

---

Lentils with Kale

Preparation time: 15 minutes

Cooking time: 20 minutes

Servings: 6

Ingredients:

- 1½ cups red lentils
- 1½ cups homemade vegetable broth

- 1½ tablespoons olive oil
- ½ cup onion, chopped
- 1 teaspoon fresh ginger, peeled and minced
- 2 garlic cloves, minced
- 1½ cups tomato, chopped
- 6 cups fresh kale, tough ends removed and chopped
- Sea salt and ground black pepper, to taste

Directions:

1. In a pan, add the broth and lentils and bring to a boil over medium-high heat.
2. Reduce the heat to low and simmer covered for about 20 minutes or until almost all the liquid is absorbed.
3. Remove from the heat and set aside still covered.
4. Meanwhile, in a large skillet, heat oil over medium heat and sauté the onion for about 5-6 minutes.
5. Add the ginger and garlic and sauté for about 1 minute.
6. Add tomatoes and kale and cook for about 4-5 minutes.
7. Stir in the lentils, salt, and black pepper then remove from heat.
8. Serve hot.

Nutrition: Calories 257 Total Fat 4.5 g Saturated Fat 0.7 g Cholesterol 0 mg Sodium 265 mg Total Carbs 39.3 g Fiber 16.5 g Sugar 2.8 g Protein 16.2 g

---

Veggie Ratatouille

Preparation time: 20 minutes

Cooking time: 45 minutes 5 minutes

Servings: 4

Ingredients:

- 6 ounces homemade tomato paste
- 3 tablespoons olive oil, divided
- ½ of an onion, chopped
- 3 tablespoons garlic, minced
- Sea salt and freshly ground black pepper, to taste
- ¾ cup filtered water
- 1 zucchini, sliced into thin circles
- 1 yellow squash, sliced into thin circles
- 1 eggplant, sliced into thin circles
- 1 red bell pepper, seeded and sliced into thin circles
- 1 yellow bell pepper, seeded and sliced into thin circles
- 1 tablespoon fresh thyme leaves, minced
- 1 tablespoon fresh lemon juice

Directions:

1. Preheat oven to 375 degrees F.

2. In a bowl, add the tomato paste, 1 tablespoon of oil, onion, garlic, salt, and black pepper and mix nicely.
3. In the bottom of a 10x10-inch baking dish, spread the tomato paste mixture evenly.
4. Arrange alternating vegetable slices starting at the outer edge of the baking dish and working concentrically towards the center.
5. Drizzle the remaining oil and lemon juice over the vegetables and sprinkle them with salt and black pepper followed by the thyme.
6. Arrange a piece of parchment paper over the vegetables.
7. Bake for about 45 minutes.
8. Serve hot.

Nutrition: Calories 206 Total Fat 11.4 g Saturated Fat 1.6 g Cholesterol 0 mg Sodium 118 mg Total Carbs 54 g Fiber 26.4 g Sugar 14.1 g Protein 5.4 g

---

Baked Beans

Preparation time: 15 minutes

Cooking time: 2 hours 5 minutes

Servings: 4

Ingredients:

- ¼ pound dry lima beans, soaked overnight and drained
- ¼ pound dry red kidney beans, soaked overnight and drained
- 1¼ tablespoons olive oil
- 1 small yellow onion, chopped
- 4 garlic cloves, minced
- 1 teaspoon dried thyme, crushed
- ½ teaspoon ground cumin
- ½ teaspoon red pepper flakes, crushed
- ¼ teaspoon smoked paprika
- 1 tablespoon fresh lemon juice
- 1 cup homemade tomato sauce
- 1 cup homemade vegetable broth
- Sea salt and freshly ground black pepper, to taste

Directions:

1. Add the beans to a large pan of boiling water and bring back to a boil.
2. Reduce the heat to low.
3. Cover the pan and cook for about 1 hour.
4. Drain the beans well.
5. Preheat the oven to 325 degrees F.
6. In a large oven-proof pan, heat the oil over medium heat and sauté the onion for about 4 minutes.
7. Add the garlic, thyme, and spices and sauté for about 1 minute.
8. Stir in the cooked beans and remaining **Ingredients:** and immediately remove from the heat.
9. Cover the pan and bake in oven for about 1 hour.
10. Serve hot.

Nutrition: Calories 270 Total Fat 13 g Saturated Fat 1.9 g Cholesterol 0 mg Sodium 433 mg Total Carbs 29.5 g Fiber 7.4 g Sugar 4.1 g Protein 10.6 g

---

<u>Barley Pilaf</u>

Preparation time: 20 minutes

Cooking time: 1 hour 5 minutes 25 minutes

Servings: 4

Ingredients:

- ½ cup pearl barley
- 1 cup vegetable broth
- 2 tablespoons vegetable oil, divided
- 2 garlic cloves, minced
- ½ cup white onion, chopped
- ½ cup green olives, sliced
- ½ cup green bell pepper, seeded and chopped
- ½ cup red bell pepper, seeded and chopped
- 2 tablespoons fresh cilantro, chopped
- 2 tablespoons fresh mint leaves, chopped
- 1 tablespoon tamari

Directions:

1. In a pan, add the barley and broth over medium-high heat and cook until boiling.
2. Immediately, reduce the heat to low and simmer covered for about 45 minutes or until all the liquid is evaporated.
3. In a large skillet, heat 1 tablespoon of the oil over medium-high heat and sauté the garlic for about 30 seconds.
4. Stir in the cooked barley and cook for about 3 minutes.
5. Remove from the heat and set aside.
6. In another skillet, heat the remaining oil over medium heat and sauté the onion for about 7 minutes.
7. Add the olives and bell peppers and stir fry for about 3 minutes.
8. Stir in remaining Ingredients: and cook for about 3 minutes.
9. Stir in the barley mixture and cook for about 3 minutes.
10. Serve hot.

Nutrition: Calories 204 Total Fat 10.1 g Saturated Fat 1.5 g Cholesterol 0 mg Sodium 572 mg Total Carbs 25.3 g Fiber 4.9 g Sugar 2.6 g Protein 4.8 g

Vegetable and Salmon Kebabs

Ingredients:

- 4 wooden skewers
- Pepper (.25 tsp.)
- Salt (.5 tsp.)
- Minced garlic cloves (1)
- Olive oil (1 Tbsp.)
- Quartered sweet onion (.5)
- Sliced yellow pepper (1)
- Cherry tomatoes (12)
- Chopped zucchini (1)
- Salmon (6 oz.)
- For the pest sauce
- Pepper (.5 tsp.)
- Salt (1 tsp.)
- Olive oil (.25 c.)
- Pumpkin seeds (.25 c.)
- Basil leaves (.5 c.)
- Minced garlic clove (1)
- Spinach (1 c.)
- Juiced lemon (1)

Directions:

1. Take out the skewers and thread the vegetables and salmon on them in the pattern that you want.
2. Add these to a baking tray and then brush on the pepper, garlic, salt, and olive oil.
3. Turn on the oven and give it time to heat up to 400 degrees. Add the skewers into the oven and bake for a bit.
4. After 20 minutes, see if the fish is cooked through and then set to the side to cool down.
5. Bring out your blender and place all of the Ingredients: for the pesto sauce inside. Add in more oil if it is needed.
6. Drizzle the pesto sauce over your salmon skewers before serving.

Coconut Curry with Vegetables

Ingredients:

- Chopped cilantro (3 Tbsp.)
- Curry powder (2 tsp.)
- Salt (1 tsp.)
- Water (.33 c.)
- Coconut milk (1 c.)
- Diced tomato (1)
- Firm tofu, sliced (8 oz.)
- Green beans (.25 lb.)
- Cubed eggplant (.5 c.)
- Yellow bell pepper sliced (1)
- Cubed zucchini (2)
- Diced yellow onion (.5)
- Coconut oil (2 Tbsp.)

Directions:

1. Bring out a skillet and heat up the coconut oil on it. After the oil is warm, add in the beans, eggplant, bell pepper, zucchini, ginger, and onion.

2. Cook these for five minutes, and then add in the tomatoes and tofu. Stir around to cook a bit longer.
3. After another 5 minutes, add in the curry powder, salt, water, and coconut milk. Let it simmer for a bit.
4. Ten minutes later, the dish is ready. Stir in the cilantro and enjoy!

Loaded Spaghetti Squash

Ingredients:

- Lemon zest (.5 tsp.)
- Torn basil leaves (1 c.)
- Salt (.5 tsp.)
- Oregano (.5 tsp.)
- Brown or green lentils, cooked (1 c.)
- Diced tomatoes (6)
- Minced garlic cloves (1)
- Chopped leek (1)
- Olive oil (1.5 Tbsp.)
- Sliced spaghetti squash (1)

Directions:

1. Turn on the oven and give it some time to heat up to 375 degrees. While that is warming up, add a bit of oil on each half of the spaghetti squash and then place these face down on a baking tray that is lined with parchment paper.
2. Add the squash to the oven and let it bake until it has time to be tender. After half an hour, the dish should be done.
3. While that is cooking, heat up the rest of the oil in a skillet. Add in the tomatoes, garlic, and leak.
4. After eight minutes, you can add in the dried oregano and the lentils, cooking for an additional 5 minutes.
5. When the squash is done, take it out of the oven and use a fork to separate out the flesh.
6. Add the lentil and vegetable mixture to this flesh and combine.
7. Top with the olive oil, lemon zest, and torn basil leaves before serving.

Spicy Pasta

Ingredients:

- Torn basil leaves (1 c.)
- Crushed pepper (1 tsp.)
- Salt (1 tsp.)
- Diced chili pepper (1)
- Sliced black olives (.5 c.)
- Diced zucchini (.5)

- Diced sun-dried tomatoes (.5 c.)
- Diced cherry tomatoes (2 c.)
- Diced carrot (1)
- Diced celery stalks (1)
- Diced shallot (1)
- Minced garlic cloves (1)
- Olive oil (3 Tbsp.)
- Spelt pasta (8 oz.)

Directions:

1. Use the instructions on the package to cook up the spelt noodles. Drain out the water and leave to the side.
2. Add some oil to a skillet before cooking the shallot, carrot, celery, and garlic until they are soft.
3. After eight minutes, toss in the zucchini, sun-dried tomatoes, cherry tomatoes, pepper, salt, chili pepper, and olives.
4. When this is done, toss the pasta into the pan and combine well. Move over to a serving plate and top with some basil leaves before serving.

Stuffed Peppers

Ingredients:

- Bell peppers, tops cut off (2)
- Crushed pepper (1 tsp.)
- Salt (1 tsp.)
- Chopped cilantro (1 Tbsp.)
- Juiced lime (.5)
- Chili powder (1 tsp.)
- Cumin (1 tsp.)
- Olive oil (2 Tbsp.)
- Diced avocado (.5)
- Diced cucumber (1)
- Diced red bell pepper (1)
- Cooked green lentils (.5 c.)
- Cooked quinoa (1 c.)

Directions:

1. Bring out a bowl and combine together the avocado, cucumber, diced bell pepper, lentil, and quinoa.
2. In another bowl, whisk together the salt, cilantro, lime juice, chili, cumin, pepper, and olive oil.
3. Pour this mixture over the lentil and quinoa mixture and stir. Use this mixture to stuff each of the peppers before serving.

Baba Ganoush Pasta

Ingredients:

- Chopped parsley (.25 c.)
- Cayenne pepper (1 pinch)
- Salt (.5 tsp.)
- Vegetable stock (1 c.)
- Chopped chili pepper (1)
- Minced garlic clove (1)
- Chopped onion (1)
- Cubed red bell pepper (.5)
- Cubed zucchini (1)
- Cubed eggplant (1)
- Olive oil (1 Tbsp.)
- Spelt pasta (6 oz.)

Directions:

1. Follow the Directions: on the package to cook up the spelt pasta, and then set it to the side.
2. Heat up some oil in a skillet, and when the oil is ready, add in the chili pepper, garlic, onion, pepper, zucchini, and eggplant to the skillet.
3. After 6 minutes of cooking, add in the vegetable stock and let it cook for another 5 minutes or until warm.
4. Take this from the oven and give it a few minutes to cool down before adding into the blender. Mix until nice and smooth.
5. Add the sauce back to your skillet and season with some of the pepper and salt. Toss in the cooked pasta and sprinkle on the parsley before serving.

Cheesy Broccoli Bowl

Ingredients:

- Crushed black pepper (.5 tsp.)
- Salt (.5 tsp.)
- Nutritional yeast (.24 c.)
- Lemon juice (1 Tbsp.)
- Cooked broccoli florets (4 c.)
- Cooked quinoa (1 c.)
- Olive oil (1 tsp.)

Directions:

1. To start this recipe, bring out a skillet and add in the oil, broccoli, and cooked quinoa.
2. After five minutes, this should be nice and warm so add in the pepper, salt, nutritional yeast, and lemon juice.
3. Take the dish off the heat and then serve warm.

Green Bean and Lentil Salad

Ingredients:

- Scallion (2 Tbsp.)
- Apple cider vinegar (.25 c.)
- Sliced green beans (2 c.)
- Halved cherry tomatoes (1 c.)
- Cooked green lentils (2 c.)
- Pesto Sauce
- Salt (1 tsp.)
- Olive oil (.25 c.)
- Chopped garlic clove (1)
- Pine nuts (2 Tbsp.)
- Spinach (.5 c.)
- Basil leaves (.75 c.)

Directions:

1. Bring out the food processor and add in all of the Ingredients: for the pesto sauce to make them creamy and smooth.
2. In another bowl, combine together the vinegar, green beans, tomatoes, lentils, and the scallions.
3. Drizzle the pesto sauce over the mixture in the bowl, toss around to coat, and then serve.

Vegetable Minestrone

Ingredients:

- Spinach (1 c.)
- Basil (1 c.)
- Pepper (1 tsp.)
- Salt (2 tsp.)
- Oregano (1 Tbsp.)
- Diced tomatoes (1 c.)
- Vegetable stock (1 c.)
- Kidney beans (.5 c.)
- Minced garlic clove (1)
- Shallot (1)
- Diced carrot (.5 c.)
- Cubed zucchini (.5 c.)
- Cubed butternut squash (.5 c.)
- Cubed eggplant (.5 c.)
- Olive oil (1 Tbsp.)

Directions:

1. Bring out a bit stock pot and heat up the olive oil inside. When the oil is warm, add the garlic, shallot, carrot, zucchini, squash, and eggplant to the pot.
2. After five minutes for those to cook, add in the salt, oregano, diced tomatoes, stock, kidney beans, and pepper.
3. Let these Ingredients: simmer together for ten more minutes, adding in more spices if you would like.
4. Stir in the spinach and basil right before serving and enjoy.

Southwest Burger

Ingredients:

- Sliced avocado (1)
- Lettuce leaves, Bibb (2)
- Arugula (1 c.)
- Dijon mustard (1 Tbsp.)
- Crushed walnuts (1 Tbsp.)
- Nutritional yeast (1 Tbsp.)
- Firm tofu (4 oz.)
- Crushed black pepper (.5 tsp.)
- Cayenne pepper (.5 tsp.)
- Ground cumin (1 tsp.)
- Salt (1 tsp.)
- Diced carrot (1)
- Diced green bell pepper (1 c.)
- Diced yellow onion (5.)
- Olive oil (1 Tbsp.)

Directions:

1. Heat up some oil in a skillet. When the oil is warm, add in the onion, pepper, cayenne, cumin, salt, carrot, and bell pepper.
2. After five minutes, the vegetables should be soft. Pour them into a bowl and let them cool down.
3. Grate the tofu over the bowl and then add in the Dijon mustard, walnuts, and nutritional yeast. Combine this well and shape into two burgers.
4. Turn on the oven and let it heat up to 400 degrees. Add the burgers on a baking tray that has been lined with paper, and then add to the oven.
5. After half an hour, the burgers should be done. Take them out of the oven and give them time to cool before topping with some avocado and serving.

Zucchini Rolls with Red Sauce

Ingredients:

- Basil leaves (15)
- Sliced zucchinis (2)
- Water (.75 c.)
- Dried oregano (1 tsp.)
- Salt (1 tsp.)
- Diced red bell pepper (1)
- Diced Roma tomatoes (3)
- Chopped yellow onion (1)
- Olive oil (1 Tbsp.)
- Basil Filling
- Chopped basil (1 handful)
- Nutmeg (.25 tsp.)
- Crushed pepper (.25 tsp.)
- Salt (.5 tsp.)
- Nutritional yeast (1 Tbsp.)
- Water (3 Tbsp.)
- Juiced lemon (1)
- Soaked cashews (1 c.)

Directions:

1. Bring out a skillet and heat up some oil inside. Add in the oregano, salt, bell pepper, tomato, and onion to make your red veggie mixture.
2. Cook for a few minutes to make the vegetables soft, and then add in some water. Let this simmer for a bit.
3. After ten minutes, take the skillet from the heat and give the vegetable mixture some time to cool down.
4. Move over to the blender and then blend until smooth.
5. Now, work on the cashew filling. Clean out the food processor and add in all the Ingredients: until they are smooth. This can take a bit so be patient to get it done.
6. Place the ribbons of zucchini on a platter in front of you and split up the filling between each one. Roll up each ribbon tightly and then add to a baking dish with the red veggie mixture out on the bottom.
7. Top each of these rolls with the rest of the red veggie mixture and add to the oven that is heated to 375 degrees.
8. After 15 minutes, take the baking dish out of the oven and let the dish cool down. Before serving, top on the basil leaves and enjoy.

Meatless Taco Wraps

Ingredients:

- Sliced avocado (.5)
- Romaine leaves (4)
- Water (.25 c.)
- Salt (.5 tsp.)
- Cumin (.5 tsp.)
- Chili powder (.5 tsp.)
- Smoked paprika (.5 tsp.)
- Minced garlic clove (1)
- Tomato paste (1 Tbsp.)
- Toasted walnuts (.5 c.)
- Cooked brown lentils (1.5 c.)
- For the salsa
- Crushed pepper (.5 tsp.)
- Salt (.5 tsp.)
- Apple cider vinegar (1 Tbsp.)
- Chopped cilantro (3 Tbsp.)
- Diced green bell pepper (.5 c.)
- Diced red bell pepper (.5 c.)
- Diced mango (.5 c.)

Directions:

1. Start out with the salsa. Do this by adding all of the Ingredients: into a bowl and stirring around to combine. Let it marinate for a bit while you work on your taco "meat."

2. Bring out the food processor and pulse together the water, salt, cumin, chili powder, paprika, garlic, tomato paste, walnuts, and lentils. You want this to still be a bit crumbly when you are done.
3. Place the walnut and lentil mixture into each romaine lettuce leaf, and then top with the salsa and the slices of avocado before serving.

Sesame and Quinoa Pilaf

Ingredients:

- Cooked green lentils (1 c.)
- Broth or water (1 c.)
- Quinoa (.5 c.)
- Minced garlic clove (1)
- Diced green bell pepper (.5 c.)
- Diced celery stalk (1)
- Sliced shallot (1)
- Crushed pepper (2 tsp.)
- Salt (2 tsp.)
- Olive oil (2 Tbsp.)
- Sliced carrots (2)
- Trimmed and sliced green beans (1 c.)
- For the dressing
- Black sesame seeds (2 Tbsp.)
- Rice vinegar (.25 c.)
- Tamari (.25 c.)
- Red chili flakes (.5 tsp.)
- Lemon zest (1 tsp.)
- Grated ginger (1 tsp.)
- Toasted sesame oil (2 tsp.)
- Avocado oil (.33 c.)

Directions:

1. Add the carrots and green beans onto some parchment paper on a baking tray. Drizzle the pepper, salt, and a tablespoon of the olive oil on top.
2. Add to the broiler of the oven and cook until they are browned. This will take about five minutes.
3. After that is done, take out a pot and add in the garlic, bell pepper, celery, shallot, and the rest of the oil inside.
4. Cook the Ingredients: for five minutes before adding in the quinoa and stirring to cook a bit longer.
5. Now, add in the water or the broth and bring to a boil. Let it simmer for a bit until the liquid is all gone.
6. Now, you can make the dressing. To do this, whisk together all of the Ingredients: in a bowl to combine.
7. When it is time to assemble, mix together the quinoa and lentils. Season with some pepper and salt and then top with the carrot and bean mixture before drizzling the dressing over the whole thing.

Blackened Salmon with Fruit Salsa

Ingredients:

- Mixed greens (4 c.)
- Olive oil (1 Tbsp.)
- Crushed pepper (.25 tsp.)
- Salt (.25 tsp.)
- Chili powder (.5 tsp.)
- Garlic powder (1 tsp.)
- Cayenne pepper (1 tsp.)
- Salmon (8 oz.)
- To make the salsa
- Salt
- Chopped cilantro (1 Tbsp.)
- Juiced and zested lime (1)
- Diced pineapple (.5 c.)
- Diced mango (.5 c.)
- Diced green bell pepper (.5)

Directions:

1. Start this recipe by making the mango pineapple salsa. Add all of the Ingredients: into a bowl and stir to combine. Set aside for now.
2. In another bowl, combine together the pepper, salt, chili powder, garlic powder, and cayenne. Place this mixture out on a flat plate to use in a moment.
3. Heat up a skillet on the stove on medium heat. Brush the olive oil all over the salmon fillet before adding the flesh side to the spice mixture on your plate.
4. Add the flesh side to the pan and let it cook. After five minutes, flip the fish over and cook a bit longer until the fish is all done.
5. Serve the fish with the mixed greens that you chose along with some of the salsa on top.

Arugula Salad with Shrimp

Ingredients:

- Crushed black pepper (.5 tsp.)
- Salt (.5 tsp.)
- Chopped parsley (1 Tbsp.)
- Minced garlic clove (1)
- Olive oil (2 Tbsp.)
- Juiced lemon (.5)
- Shrimp (10)
- For the salad
- Toasted pine nuts (2 tsp.)
- Salt (1 tsp.)
- Olive oil (2 Tbsp.)
- Juiced lemon (.5)
- Apple cider vinegar (2 Tbsp.)
- Halved cherry tomatoes (10)
- Arugula (4 c.)

Directions:

1. Take out a bowl and add in the pepper, parsley, salt, garlic, olive oil, lemon juice, and shrimp inside. Place into the fridge to marinate for fifteen minutes or more.
2. When you are ready, take out a skillet and heat it up. Add the prepared shrimp inside and cook for a bit on each side until the shrimp is all cooked through.
3. Now, it is time to make the salad. Bring out a big salad bowl and combine together all of the Ingredients: for the salad together.
4. Add the shrimp on top of the salad and then serve warm.

Easy Pizza

Ingredients:

- Lemon juice (1 tsp.)
- Salt (1 tsp.)
- Nutritional yeast (2 Tbsp.)
- Olive oil (2 tsp.)
- Arugula (1 c.)
- Sliced tomato (1)
- Sliced avocado (1)
- For the dough
- Dried basil (1 tsp.)
- Dried oregano (1 tsp.)
- Pepper (1 tsp.)
- Salt (1 tsp.)
- Olive oil (4 Tbsp.)
- Minced garlic clove (1)
- Ground flaxseeds (.33 c.)
- Sunflower seeds, soaked (1.25 c.)

Directions:

1. Bring out a blender and pulse the sunflower seeds a few times. Then add them into a big bowl along with the basil, oregano, salt, pepper, olive oil, garlic, and flaxseed flour.
2. Knead this mixture together until you get a nice dough to form. You can add in some more water if needed.
3. Roll the dough out into the shape of a pizza. Add some parchment paper to your baking tray and put the dough on top.
4. Heat your oven to the lowest temperature that it allows and then place the baking tray inside to dehydrate the dough. Give this about 12 hours to finish up.
5. When the dough is ready, you can layer on the tomato slices and avocado on the crust.
6. Toss the arugula into a small bowl with the lemon juice, salt, nutritional yeast, and olive oil. Place this on top of the pizza and serve the whole thing right away.

Spelt Bread

Servings: 1 loaf

Ingredients:

- 3/4 - 1 cup alkaline water
- ½ cup unsweetened hemp milk
- 3 tablespoons avocado oil
- 1 tablespoon agave nectar
- 1 ½ teaspoons fine sea salt
- 4 cups spelt flour+½ cup more for kneading

Directions:

1. Preheat the oven to 375 degrees F. Meanwhile, combine all the dry contents in a bowl.
2. Add in ¾ cup of water, hemp milk and avocado oil until fully blended to create a soft batter.
3. In case the batter seems quite stiff, add a few tablespoons of alkaline water until you get a soft mixture. And if too wet, add a few more tablespoons of spelt flour, mixing after each spoonful until the dough holds well.
4. Cover the working surface with approximately ½ cup of spelt flour. Then knead the dough on the floured surface and roll it to coat with the flour.
5. Knead the dough for another 2 or 3 minutes, and add a little more spelt in each addition until you get unified ball that can spring back when prodded.
6. At this point, get a parchment paper and line a standard loaf pan across its widths. Get some avocado oil and also grease the ends of the pan.
7. Turn the dough into the prepared loaf pan and pat it to well distribute in the pan. Score the top of the loaf using a sharp knife, lengthwise.
8. Finally bake the bread until cooked through, or for approximately 45 minutes.
9. Remove it from the oven and insert a toothpick into the center of the bread. If the toothpick or thin sharp knife doesn't come out clean, bake for an additional 5 to 10 minutes.
10. Allow the loaf to cool fully in the pan and then slice it. Serve this with some soup and top it with avocado. Also sprinkle some smoked paprika and lemon if you like it.
11. Nutritional information for (2 lb.) loaf of bread: Calories: 2785 Fat: 61.27g Carbohydrates: 494.2g Protein: 105g

Green Goddess Bowl with Avocado Dressing

Servings: 4

Ingredients:

- For salad:
- 2 tablespoons hemp seeds
- 1/3 cup cherry tomatoes, halved
- ½ cup kelp noodles, soaked and drained
- ½ zucchini
- 3 cups kale, chopped
- Avocado dressing:
- Dash cayenne pepper
- 1 tablespoons extra virgin olive oil
- ¼ teaspoon sea salt
- 1 cup filtered water
- 2 limes, fresh squeezed
- 1 tablespoons dried sage
- 1 avocado
- Tahini Lemon Dressing:
- 1 tablespoons extra virgin olive oil
- ¾ teaspoon sea salt
- 1 fennel bulb
- ½ fresh squeezed lemon
- ½ cup filtered water
- ¼ cup tahini, sesame butter
- Cayenne pepper to taste

Directions:

1. First make noodles of the zucchini using a spiralizer.
2. Then lightly steam kale for approximately 4 minutes, and set aside.
3. Combine kelp noodles with zucchini noodles and toss together with the avocado cumin dressing.
4. Now add in the cherry tomatoes and toss well. Plate the steamed broccoli and kale and season with the tahini dressing.
5. Serve the kale with tomatoes and noodles sprinkled with some hemp seeds.
6. Nutritional information per (8 oz.) serving: Calories: 324 Fat: 24.9g Carbohydrates: 24.13g Protein: 7.04g

Asian Sesame Dressing and Noodles

Servings: 2

Ingredients:

- 1 bag Kelp Noodles or 1 Zucchini to make noodles
- 1 tablespoon raw sesame seeds, topping
- 1 scallion, chopped
- Parsnip, optional
- Sliced red bell pepper, optional
- For dressing:
- 1 fennel bulb, chopped
- ½ teaspoon lemon, fresh squeezed

- ½ teaspoon agave sugar
- 2 tablespoons tahini, sesame butter

Directions:

1. With a vegetable peeler or spiralizer, cut out noodle-sized strips or use 1 bag of kelp noodles.
2. Mix all the Ingredients: for dressing in a bowl, and mix well with a spoon. If using kelp noodles, put them in warm water for about 10 minutes to soften them.
3. Pour the sesame dressing on the scallions and noodles, and mix well. Top with sesame if you like it and enjoy.
4. Nutritional information per (9 oz.) serving: Calories: 462 Fat: 11.23g Carbohydrates: 77.34g Protein: 14.7g

---

Instant Alkaline Sushi Roll Ups

Servings: 2

Ingredients:

- For the Dip/Hummus
- 1 fennel bulb
- A glug of olive oil
- 1 pinch of dried sage
- 1 tablespoons tahini
- A handful of walnuts
- 100g of chickpeas/garbanzos from a can, drained
- Pinch of Himalayan salt
- Juice of 1/2 lemon
- For the Roll-Ups
- 1 capsicum sliced into matchsticks
- 1 small bunch culantro
- 1 avocado, peeled and sliced
- 1 cucumber, sliced into matchsticks
- 1 parsnips, sliced into matchsticks
- 2 medium zucchini/courgettes

Directions:

1. In a blender or food processor, puree all the Ingredients: for the hummus. Add a bit of lemon and olive oil in equal amounts until you get desired consistency.
2. To make the alkaline rolls up, first chop the zucchini or courgettes into thin long strips using a vegetable peeler.
3. Lay individual zucchini strip out and spread a generous amount of almond hummus onto the zucchini strip.
4. Now add little amounts of avocado, colander and the matchsticks of veggies.
5. Top with some sesame seeds and then serve.
6. Nutritional information per (16 oz.) serving: Calories: 743 Fat: 51.69g Carbohydrates: 50.95g Protein: 31.77g

Quinoa Stuffed Spaghetti Squash

Servings: 2

Ingredients:

- 1 teaspoon minced ginger
- 2 teaspoon dried thyme
- 1 and 1/2 cup cooked quinoa
- 1/4 cup chopped walnuts
- 2 spring onions, white part, sliced
- 1 orange or red bell pepper
- 1 medium shallot
- 1 cup steamed green peas
- 2 tablespoons coconut oil
- 1 big or two smaller spaghetti squashes
- Sea salt and cayenne pepper to taste

Directions:

1. Preheat the oven to 400 degrees F.
2. Then clean the squashes, slice in half and then discard the seeds. Bake the squash for approximately 40 minutes or until tender.
3. Meanwhile, in a skillet, heat a tablespoon of coconut oil and cook bell pepper and chopped shallots until soft.
4. Then add in cooked quinoa, green peas, spices and walnuts and cook until warmed through. Season the mixture with salt and pepper.
5. At this point, divide the mixture between the squash and bake until cooked through, or for about 5 to 8 minutes.
6. Remove from heat and serve the stuffed spaghetti squash with fresh greens such as kale.
7. Nutritional information per (12 oz.) serving: Calories: 429 Fat: 22.96g Carbohydrates: 48.43g Protein: 13.18g

---

Spelt Pasta with Spicy Eggplant Sauce

Servings: 2

Ingredients:

- Some cold-pressed extra virgin olive oil
- 1 pinch of cayenne pepper
- 1/2 teaspoon organic sea salt
- 1 handful of fresh basil
- 1 cup vegetable stock
- 1 small chili
- 1 fennel bulb
- 1 medium-sized onion
- 1 fresh red bell pepper
- 1 fresh eggplant
- 1 cup spelt pasta

Directions:

1. Cook the spelt pasta according to package Directions:.
2. Meanwhile cut the bell pepper and eggplant into cubes and then chop basil, fennel bulb, onion and chili into small pieces.
3. In a pan, heat some olive oil and then stir-fry fennel bulb and onions for a few minutes.
4. Add pepper cubes and eggplant along with the chili and now cook for additional 2 to 3 minutes.
5. At this point dissolve the veggie stock in 1 cup alkaline water then add the mixture to the pan.
6. Simmer the contents, stirring a few times, for approximately 10 minutes on low heat.
7. Add basil and season with some pepper and salt. Spoon the sauce over the spelt pasta and enjoy!
8. Nutritional information per (16 oz.) serving: Calories: 651 Fat: 14.86g Carbohydrates: 121.99g Protein: 25.6g

---

Sesame Kale with Garbanzo Beans

Servings: 2

Ingredients:

- 1 tablespoon sesame oil
- 1 tablespoon sesame seeds
- 2 tablespoons lemon juice
- 15 oz. garbanzo beans
- 1 fennel bulb, chopped
- 1 bunch green onions, sliced thin
- 2 tablespoons olive oil
- Salt to taste
- 1 bunch of kale

Directions:

1. Start by cutting the kale. Tear the leaves from the stem, roll them up and chop them into tiny pieces.
2. Add some olive oil into a skillet and then sauté green onions and fennel on low heat setting for about 1 minute.
3. Add in the beans and sauté for a further 4 to 5 minutes. Add in the kale, lemon juice and season with some salt.
4. Cook until the kale has reduced in size. Serve the kale, drizzle some sesame oil and some sesame seeds.
5. Nutritional information per (14 oz.) serving: Calories: 313 Fat: 24.41g Carbohydrates: 23.22g Protein: 6.37g

Alkaline Vegan Meatloaf

Servings: 1 loaf

Ingredients:

- 1 cup prepared wild rice
- 1/2 cup homemade tomato sauce, divided
- 1/2 cup chopped yellow or white onion, divided
- 1/2 cup chopped green bell pepper, divided
- 1 shallot, roughly chopped
- 2 cups mixed mushrooms, roughly chopped
- 1/4 teaspoon cloves
- 1/2 teaspoon ginger
- 1/2 teaspoon tarragon
- 1 teaspoon thyme
- 1 teaspoon sage
- 1 tablespoons sea salt
- 1 tablespoons onion powder
- 1 cup garbanzo flour or spelt flour
- 1.5 cups breadcrumbs (made of spelt flour)
- 2 cups cooked chickpeas
- Cayenne to taste

Directions:

1. Clean and dry the wild rice as required. Prepare the chickpeas as well and set them aside.
2. Mix together garbanzo flour or spelt flour with bread crumbs and set the mixture aside.
3. Chop the green peppers and the onions and place half of each of them to the side.
4. Now chop the shallots and mushrooms and add them to a food processor; along with chickpeas, half of the onion, half of the green peppers and spices.
5. Pulse the mixture until fully incorporated. Then add in 2 tablespoons of tomato sauce and the wild rice, and continue to blend until you obtain coarse paste.
6. Move the mixture to a mixing bowl large enough to accommodate the remaining flour, bread crumbs, onion and green pepper. Mix until blended.
7. At this point, put the mixture in a greased pan and cover with the remaining tomato sauce.
8. Bake in a preheated oven at 350 degrees F for approximately 60 to 70 minutes- keeping an eye on the top so as not to burn.
9. Then remove from the oven and allow to cool down for about 30 minutes or so. Serve with some sauce and vegetables and enjoy.
10. Nutritional Information Per (2 lb.) Serving: Calories: 265 Carbs: 48.0g Protein: 13.15g Fat: 2.96g

Alkaline Pizza Crust

Servings: 4

Ingredients:

- 1 cup spring water
- 2 teaspoons grapeseed oil
- 2 teaspoons agave
- 1 teaspoon sea salt
- 2 teaspoons sesame seeds
- 1 teaspoon oregano
- 1 teaspoon onion powder
- 1 1/2 cups spelt flour
- Toppings (Optional)
- Cherry tomatoes
- Onions

Directions:

1. First, preheat the oven to 400 degrees F.
2. In a medium-sized bowl, mix all the Ingredients: along with ½ cup of water.
3. Add more water in little amounts until you have dough that rolls into a ball, or add extra flour if the dough appears runny.
4. Coat a baking sheet with some oil, and add some flour to your hands.
5. Now roll out the thick dough into the baking sheet and brush the top with extra grapeseed oil.
6. Using a fork, poke a few holes on the dough and bake it in the preheated oven for approximately 10 to 15 minutes.
7. Meanwhile start making the avocado pizza sauce. *** (recipe included)
8. Once the crust is cooked through, add the pizza sauce and whatever alkaline friendly toppings you would like such as cherry tomatoes, onions etc. to the crust
9. Bake until well cooked, or for another 15 to 20 minutes.

For Pizza Sauce

Ingredients:

- 1/2 teaspoon oregano
- 1/2 teaspoon sea salt
- 1/2 teaspoon onion powder
- 2 tablespoons chopped onion
- 1 avocado
- Pinch of basil

Directions:

1. To make the avocado pizza sauce, first cut the avocado down the middle, discard the pit and then scrap the avocado meat into a food processor.
2. Add all other sauce Ingredients: and process until smooth or for about 3 minutes or so. Scrap the inside of the food processor once needed.
3. Nutritional Information Per (7 oz.) Serving Calories: 1013 Carbs: 188.0g Protein: 39.25g Fat: 18.5g

Alkaline Electric Vegan "Ribs"

Servings: 1 serving

Ingredients:

- Grapeseed oil
- 1/2 teaspoon cayenne
- 1 teaspoon onion powder
- 1 teaspoon sea salt
- 1/4 cup spring water
- 2 Portobello mushrooms
- 1/2 cup Alkaline Barbecue Sauce
- For Alkaline Electric Barbecue Sauce
- Servings: about 8-10 ounces

- 1/8 teaspoon cloves
- 1/4 teaspoon cayenne powder
- 1/2 teaspoon ground ginger
- 2 teaspoon onion powder
- 2 teaspoon smoked sea salt/sea salt
- 1/4 cup white onions, chopped
- 1/4 cup date sugar
- 2 tablespoons agave
- 6 cherry tomatoes

Directions:

1. First, remove the gills from the bottom of individual mushroom caps and then slice the Portobello approximately ½ inch apart.
2. Put the sauce Ingredients: in a blender and puree until smooth.
3. Add the sliced mushrooms to a container along with water, large amounts of barbeque sauce and the seasoning.
4. Cover the mixture and then keep it chilled for approximately 6 to 8 hours. Ensure that you flip over at regular intervals of 2 hours.
5. Pick a skewer and push about 3 Portobello mushrooms around the middle, then pick another skewer and repeat. If any of the mushroom slices break, reserve them as rib-lets.
6. Brush a griddle with grapeseed oil and then cook the ribs over medium heat for around 12 to 15 minutes. Remember to flip regularly, after every 3 minutes.
7. Brush with additional sauce after a few flips and serve with your favorite alkaline-friendly dish.
8. Nutritional Information Per (6 oz.) Serving Calories: 149 Carbs: 36.27 g Protein: 2.42 g Fat: 0.7g

Walnut Meat

Servings: 6

Ingredients:

- 1/2 cup fresh thyme, chopped
- 1/2 teaspoon sea salt
- 1 pinch dried basil
- 1 small red onion, chopped
- 1 1/2 cups red bell pepper, chopped
- 4 cups soaked walnuts

Directions:

1. First, soak the walnuts in spring water for at least 4 hours, or preferably overnight.
2. Add the soaked walnuts in the food processor along with bell pepper and onions.
3. Add in salt, thyme and process on high speed setting until you achieve your preferred consistency- whether smooth or chunky.
4. Transfer the mixture to a bowl using a rubber spatula and dehydrate to make into walnut crumble or meat patties.
5. You can also add the contents to an airtight container and keep it refrigerated for a maximum of 1 week.
6. Nutritional Information Per (3 oz.) Serving Calories: 364 Carbs: 10.43g Protein: 8.55g Fat: 34.01g

---

Alkaline Electric Mushroom Cheese Steak

Servings: 4

Ingredients:

- Mushroom Mix:
- 1 teaspoon savory
- 1 teaspoon thyme
- 1 teaspoon oregano
- 1 teaspoon smoked sea salt
- 1 tablespoons onion powder
- 1 tablespoons grapeseed oil
- 1/2 cup alkaline electric "garlic" sauce
- 1 cup red bell peppers
- 1 cup green bell peppers
- 1 cup onions, sliced
- 4 portabella mushroom caps
- For Cheese:
- 1/2 teaspoon basil
- 1/2 teaspoon sea salt
- 1/2 teaspoon oregano
- 1/2 teaspoon cayenne powder
- 1 1/2 teaspoon onion powder
- 1 1/2 teaspoon hemp seeds
- 1/3 – 1/2 cup spring water
- 3/4 cup Brazil nuts, soaked

Directions:

1. First, slice the mushrooms to around 1/8th inch thick. Then in a bowl, whisk the sauce along with seasonings to prepare some marinade.
2. Toss sliced portabella mushroom caps in the marinade, and let it sit for approximately 30 minutes. Mix after about 15 minutes.
3. To make the "cheese", blend all the Ingredients: in a blender until fully incorporated.
4. Meanwhile, add grapeseed oil in a skillet over medium heat and sauté peppers and onions for about 3 to 5 minutes.
5. Then add in the marinated portabellas and sauté for 5 more minutes. Serve the cheese steak with a flatbread and enjoy.
6. Nutritional Information Per (6 oz.) Serving Calories: 253 Carbs: 15.42g Protein: 5.55g Fat: 21.17g

---

Alkaline Electric Chickpea Tofu

Servings: 2

Ingredients:

- 1 teaspoon culantro
- 1 teaspoon sea salt
- 1 cup chickpea flour
- 2 cups spring water

Directions:

1. First, line a baking dish with some parchment papers.
2. Then in a saucepan, whisk continually all the above Ingredients: on medium heat until you obtain porridge like mixture, or for around 3 to 5 minutes.
3. Pour the batter in a baking dish and smooth it out using a spatula.
4. Let it cool down until firm, or for about 30 minutes or so. You can keep it in the fridge to help fasten the process.
5. Once firm enough, put the tofu in a cutting board and slice it into bite-sized cubes.
6. Serve it as is or bake or sauté it for a few more minutes. Season as you like it and serve.
7. Nutritional Information Per (10 oz.) Serving Calories: 178 Carbs: 26.6g Protein: 10.32g Fat: 3.08g

Alkaline Electric Egg Foo Yung

Servings: 6

Ingredients:

- Grapeseed oil
- 1 cup spring water
- 1/8 teaspoon ginger powder
- 1/2 teaspoon cayenne powder
- 1 teaspoon oregano
- 1 teaspoon sea salt
- 1 teaspoon onion powder
- 1 teaspoon basil
- 3/4 cup garbanzo bean flour
- 1/2 cup red & white onion, chopped
- 1/2 cup green onions, chopped
- 1/2 cup red & green peppers, chopped
- 1 cup butternut squash, chopped
- 2 cups mushrooms, sliced
- 3 cups prepared spaghetti squash

Directions:

1. Begin by whisking the seasonings, garbanzo flour and spring water in a bowl.
2. Then add in the veggies and prepared spaghetti squash. Combine with your hands until incorporated together.
3. Using grapeseed oil, coat a large skillet well on high heat and then add ½ cup of the squash and vegetable mixture.
4. Pat down the dough into patties and cook in the hot skillet until brown, or for approximately 3 to 4 minutes on each side. Add extra oil if need be.
5. Serve the egg foo yung with fried wild rice and alkaline friendly sauce and enjoy.
6. Nutritional Information Per (6 oz.) Serving Calorie: 139 Carbs: 24.76g Protein: 6.65g Fat: 2.1g

---

Alkaline Electric Pasta Salad

Servings: 4

Ingredients:

- 1/4 cup black olives
- 1/2 cup cherry tomatoes, cut in half
- 1/2 cup onions, diced
- 1 cup zucchini/summer squash, sliced
- 1 cup red/yellow/green bell peppers, diced
- 4 cups cooked spelt pasta
- 3/4 to 1 cup alkaline electric "garlic" sauce

Directions:

1. In a large bowl, toss together all the Ingredients: until well incorporated.
2. Serve and enjoy.
3. Nutritional Information Per (10 oz.) Serving Calories: 229 Carbs: 62.8g Protein: 11.4g Fat: 2.66g

---

Mushroom "Chicken Tenders"

Servings: 6

Ingredients:

- Grapeseed oil
- 1 teaspoon ground cloves
- 1 teaspoon cayenne powder
- 2 teaspoon ginger powder
- 2 teaspoon onion powder
- 2 teaspoon sage
- 2 teaspoon sea salt
- 2 teaspoon basil
- 2 teaspoon oregano
- 1 1/2 cup spelt flour
- 1 1/2 cups spring water
- 2-6 portabella, oyster or white mushrooms

Directions:

1. First, slice the portabella, oyster or white mushrooms caps approximately half-inch apart and add them to a large bowl. You can also chop off mushrooms stems to prepare nuggets.
2. Add some grapeseed oil, water and half of individual seasonings to the bowl and let the mixture marinate for approximately 1 hour.
3. In a separate bowl, blend the rest of the seasonings along with the spelt flour and then batter the mushrooms.
4. If baking, preheat your oven to 400 degrees F. Meanwhile grease a baking sheet with grapeseed oil and then put the mushrooms on the baking sheet.
5. Bake each side until crispy, flipping once, or for approximately 15 minutes per side. Serve.
6. If using a stovetop, heat a skillet over medium high heat. Then add about 3 tablespoons of grapeseed oil to the skillet.
7. Cook the mushrooms until crispy, or for about 3 to 4 minutes per side. Be careful not to pop oil because of either high heat or liquid from the mushrooms. Enjoy!
8. Nutritional Information Per (6 oz.) Serving Calories: 276 Carbs: 49.48g Protein: 10.72g Fat: 6.5g

Margarita Pizza

Servings: 6

Ingredients:

- Crust:
- 1 1/2 cups spelt flour
- 1 cup spring water
- 1/2 teaspoon onion powder
- 1/2 teaspoon oregano
- 1/2 teaspoon sea salt
- 1/2 teaspoon basil
- Cheese:
- 1/4 teaspoon sea salt
- 1/2 teaspoon basil
- 1/2 teaspoon oregano

- 1/2 teaspoon onion powder
- 1 teaspoon lime juice
- 1/4 cup hemp milk/nut milk
- 1/2 cup spring water
- 1 cup Brazil nuts, soaked for over 2 hours
- Toppings:
- Alkaline electric tomato sauce
- Red onion, sliced
- Plum tomatoes, sliced

Directions:

1. In a medium bowl, combine all seasonings with the spelt flour and then add in half cup of water.
2. Add more water in little amounts until the dough can roll into a ball, or add more spelt flour in case you find the dough wet.
3. Roll the dough on a floured surface, in one direction as you flip and turn it after a couple of rolls. Keep adding spelt flour after flipping to keep the dough from becoming too sticky.
4. Place the dough into a baking sheet that is gently coated with oil, poking holes with a fork, and now bake in a preheated oven at 350 degrees for approximately 10 to 15 minutes.
5. Meanwhile, add all Ingredients: for cheese in a blender, and process them until smooth, or for about 1 to 2 minutes.
6. As soon as the crust is cooked through, coat it with the cheese, alkaline electric sauce and your preferred toppings. Add more cheese and sauce if you like.
7. Bake the contents on the bottom of the rack at 425 degrees F for a further 10 to 15 minutes. Enjoy!
8. Nutritional Information Per (6 oz.) Serving Calories: 322 Carbs: 34.17g Protein: 9g Fat: 18.75g

Alkaline Electric Veggie Lasagna

Servings: 6

Ingredients:

- Pasta
- Spelt Lasagna Sheets
- Tomato Sauce
- 1/2 teaspoon cayenne powder
- 2 teaspoon sea salt
- 2 teaspoons oregano
- 2 teaspoons basil
- 1 tablespoons onion powder
- 1 tablespoons agave
- 12 plum tomatoes
- "Meat" Alternative
- 1 teaspoon fennel powder
- 2 teaspoon basil
- 2 teaspoon oregano
- 1 tablespoons sea salt
- 2 tablespoons onion powder
- 1/2 cup tomato sauce
- 1 cup green, yellow, and red peppers, diced
- 1 cup onions, chopped
- 1 cup cooked chickpeas (garbanzo beans)
- 2 cups cooked spelt berries/kernels
- Brazil Nut Cheese
- 1 teaspoon basil
- 1 teaspoon oregano
- 1 teaspoon sea salt
- 1 tablespoons onion powder
- 1 tablespoon hemp seeds
- 1 cup spring water
- 2 cups soaked Brazil nuts
- Extras
- White Mushrooms
- Grapeseed Oil
- Zucchini

Directions:

1. Add the Ingredients: for tomato sauce in a blender and then process until well combined.
2. Add grapeseed oil to a saucepan with the tomato sauce and heat the sauce over medium heat. Lower the heat and simmer until the sauce has thickened, or for 2 hours, stirring regularly.
3. In a food processor, combine Ingredients: for "meat" that is garbanzo beans, spelt and the seasonings until well incorporated.
4. Lightly coat a skillet with oil and heat it over medium heat. Sauté peppers and onions for approximately 5 minutes.
5. Now add the garbanzo and spelt mixture from the food processor, and some grapeseed oil to the skillet and cook the mixture until it begins to brown, or for 10 to 12 minutes.

6. Into a blender, add in the remaining cheese Ingredients: along with a cup of water and process until blended well. If you find it too thick, add ¼ cup of spring water at a time until you get the consistency that you want.
7. Reserve a cup of tomato sauce, and then pour the rest of the sauce into the garbanzo bean and spelt mixture. Combine well.
8. Slice the zucchini and the mushrooms lengthwise. You can also make the lasagna from the zucchini in place of the spelt pasta if you like.
9. At this point, begin making the lasagna. Lightly coat the bottom of the dish with the reserved tomato sauce to ensure it doesn't stick.
10. Then lay the spelt pasta, sliced zucchini, the garbanzo/spelt mixture, alkaline cheese, white mushrooms, and the spelt pasta again.
11. Repeat this arrangement until you get 4 layers of the pasta. Then top the last layer with the garbanzo/spelt mixture and cheese.
12. Pour the rest of tomato sauce around the lasagna layers and sprinkle with some dried basil if you like.
13. Bake everything at 350 degrees F for approximately 35 to 45 minutes.
14. Then let the lasagna cool down for around 15 minutes or so and then serve.
15. Nutritional Information Per (12 oz.) Serving Calories: 575 Carbs: 60.43g Protein: 11.5g Fat: 36.17g

Stuffed Eggplant

Servings: 6

Ingredients:

- Cayenne pepper
- Sea salt
- 2 tablespoons tomato puree
- 1 teaspoon ground caraway
- 1 teaspoon of agave
- 1 cup chopped cherry tomatoes
- 1 green bell pepper, seeded and chopped
- 2 medium red onions, chopped
- 3 tablespoons chopped fresh sage/basil
- 1 fennel bulb, chopped
- 4 tablespoons olive oil, divided
- 6 slender eggplants

Directions:

1. Preheat your oven to 450 degrees F and then put a rack in the middle of the oven.
2. Line a baking sheet using a parchment paper or foil then brush with some olive oil.
3. Then remove the wide strips of the eggplant skin using a vegetable peeler. Cut the eggplants open lengthwise but don't slice completely through.

4. Now sprinkle a pinch of salt in each and then put in a colander for around 30 minutes.
5. Put them on the baking sheet and bake until the outer skins start to shrivel, in around 20 minutes. Remove from the oven and cool.
6. Meanwhile, heat 2 tablespoons of olive oil in a large skillet over medium heat and add the onions.
7. Cook for a few minutes while stirring occasionally, and then add fennel and bell pepper. Cook for about 10 minutes, or until the veggies are tender and have collapsed.
8. Season the mixture with salt and cayenne pepper then stir in parsley, tomato puree, caraway, sugar and chopped tomato.
9. Cook until fragrant, in about 5 minutes. Set aside. Lower the oven temperature to 350 degrees F.
10. In a baking dish, arrange the eggplants in a manner that each is butterflied open. Season with salt and fill with tomato and onion mixture.
11. Drizzle with the rest of olive oil, and then add two tablespoons of water to the baking dish. Bake until the eggplants are flat and the liquid in pan caramelized, in about 40-45 minutes.
12. Serve the eggplant either warm or at room temperature, preferably with pan juices drizzled over the eggplant.
13. Nutritional information per (16 oz.) serving: Calories: 272 Fat: 10.64g Carbohydrates: 44.46g Protein: 7.52g

---

Quinoa Pasta with Tomato Artichoke Sauce

Servings: 2

Ingredients:

- 2 tablespoons extra-virgin olive oil, cold-pressed
- 1 pinch of cayenne pepper
- 1/2 teaspoon sea salt, organic
- 3 tablespoons basil, fresh
- 1 teaspoon vegetable stock, yeast-free
- 1 ounce walnuts
- 1 fennel bulb
- 1 medium-sized onion
- 8 ounces artichoke hearts, fresh or frozen
- 5 ounces cherry tomatoes, fresh
- 7 ounces quinoa or spelt pasta

Directions:

1. Cook the artichoke until tender.

2. Then cook the pasta according to its package **Directions:**. As it cooks, cut the tomatoes into cubes, and then chop the basil, fennel and onion into pieces.
3. In a pan, heat 2 tablespoons of olive oil and stir-fry onions, nuts and fennel for a few minutes. Then add in the cooked artichoke hearts and tomatoes and cook for 2 minutes.
4. Scoop about 1/2 cup of water and then dissolve the vegetable stock into the water. Add into a pan. Let it simmer for 2 minutes on low heat, while stirring regularly.
5. At the end, add in basil and season with salt and cayenne pepper. To serve, pour the sauce over the pasta.
6. Nutritional information per (14 oz.) serving: Calories: 719 Fat: 26.21g Carbohydrates: 111g Protein: 23.91g

Sautéed Mushrooms

Servings: 6

Ingredients:

- 1 fennel bulb, chopped
- ½ lemons
- 1 ½ teaspoons sea salt
- 3 tablespoons olive oil, extra-virgin
- 2 tablespoons sage, chopped
- 1/4 teaspoon cayenne pepper
- 24 ounces mushrooms, fresh

Directions:

1. Submerge the mushrooms in water and swish them around to clean them thoroughly, and drain completely. Trim and slice your mushrooms to bite-sizes.
2. Place the mushrooms in a bowl and squeeze the juice from the lemon half into them. Toss to mix.
3. In a large pan, add fennel and then pour olive oil. Heat the mixture over medium-high heat until the fennel begins to sizzle; this should take about 30 seconds.
4. Now add in the mushrooms, stir, and cover. Continue cooking while stirring occasionally; say at intervals of around 4 minutes.
5. Once cooked through, remove the lid and add some salt and cayenne pepper, and continue cooking. After about 5 minutes, your mushrooms should begin to brown, and all moisture should have evaporated.
6. Now stir in the sage and then serve the delicious meal. Enjoy!
7. Nutritional information per (6 oz.) serving: Calories: 409 Fat: 7.98g Carbohydrates: 88.72g Protein: 11.41g

Alkaline Electric Flatbread

Servings: 4

Ingredients:

- 1/4 teaspoon cayenne
- 2 teaspoons onion powder
- 2 teaspoons basil
- 2 teaspoons oregano
- 1 tablespoon sea salt
- 3/4 cup spring water
- 2 tablespoons grapeseed oil
- 2 cups spelt flour

Directions:

1. Begin by combining all the seasonings and flour together until well incorporated.
2. Then add in ½ cup of water and oil and mix well until the mixture rolls into a ball.
3. Put some flour on the workspace and now knead the dough for approximately 5 minutes. Divide the dough into 6 portions.
4. Roll individual balls into 4-inch or so circles. Place the balls in a skillet and cook on medium heat until cooked through, while flipping after 3 minutes or so.
5. Serve with some curry.
6. Nutritional information per (6 oz.) serving:
7. Calories: 361 Fat: 8.18g Carbohydrates: 62.97g Protein: 12.32g

---

Alkaline Dinner Plate

Servings: 4

Ingredients:

- Kale Dish
- 1/2 cup chopped red onions
- 1/4 habanero pepper
- 2 tablespoons of agave
- Sea salt
- 1/2 cup green onions
- 1 cup chopped orange, yellow and sweet red peppers
- 2 bunches kale greens
- Pasta Dish
- 1/2 teaspoon of grapeseed oil
- 1/2 cup chopped yellow squash
- 1/4 cup chopped red and green peppers
- 1 teaspoon sea salt
- 1/4 cup chopped green and red onions
- 1 cup chopped portabella mushrooms
- 1 box Kamut pasta
- Fried Oyster Mushrooms
- Sea salt to taste
- ½ cup spelt flour
- Dash of Cayenne pepper
- ½ teaspoon onion powder

- 1/2 king oyster mushroom, large
- Avocado slices, optional

Directions:

1. Clean the kale and chop it to bite-sizes. Using grapeseed oil, gently coat the bottom of a cooking pot and add in peppers and onions.
2. Sauté the veggies for a few seconds then add kale and agave. Cook the mixture on medium heat, stirring regularly, for 30 minutes or so.
3. Now bring water in a pot to a boil and add in ½ teaspoon of oil and a teaspoon of salt. Add in kamut pasta
4. Sauté peppers, onions and portabella mushrooms in a sauce pan for a few minutes.
5. Add in the cooked kamut pasta to the veggies along with chopped squash. Mix well.
6. At this point, rinse the oyster mushrooms, season with cayenne pepper, onion powder and sea salt.
7. Coat the mushrooms with spelt flour and fry in oil. Once cooked through, remove from heat and put it on towel place to absorb extra oil.
8. Serve it while still warm.
9. Nutritional information per (12 oz.) serving: Calories: 600 Fat: 12.56g Carbohydrates: 50.94g Protein: 16.89g

---

Alkalizing Tahini Noodle Bowl

Servings: 2

Ingredients:

- Bowl
- 1 teaspoon black sesame seeds
- 1/2 avocado, sliced
- 2 green onions, chopped
- 4 kale, chopped
- 1 parsnip, shredded
- 4 leaves of romaine, chopped
- 1 yellow zucchini, spiralized
- Dressing
- 1 teaspoon agave or any other liquid sweetener
- 2 tablespoons lemon juice
- 1 tablespoon tahini
- Dash of salt

Directions:

1. Slice, chop and shred the vegetables as indicated above, add them in a bowl.
2. Add all Ingredients: for dressing in another small bowl and whisk until fully combined.
3. Pour the dressing over the vegetables, and garnish with sesame seeds.
4. Nutritional information per (8 oz.) serving: Calories: 209 Fat: 14.5g Carbohydrates: 22.07g Protein: 5.49g

PH Balancing Alkaline Salad

Servings: 4

Ingredients:

- 1 tablespoon sesame seeds
- 1 tablespoon diced spring onion
- 1/4 cup chopped culantro
- 1/2 cup chopped alfalfa sprouts
- 1/2 cup chopped snow pea sprouts
- 1/2 avocado
- 5 red radishes
- 1 cup chopped arugula
- 10 green beans
- Dressing
- 1 teaspoon mustard greens
- 1 tablespoons olive oil
- 1 tablespoon of lemon juice
- 1/4 teaspoon Celtic sea salt
- Cayenne pepper, to taste

Directions:

1. Mix all the Ingredients: for dressing in a large bowl until blended.
2. Wash and cut the green beans edges.
3. Add the green beans to a saucepan and add in enough water to almost cover them. Cook on low heat until almost tender, or for approximately 3 minutes.
4. Remove the green beans from heat and let them drain out. Then chop the green beans into 1-inch pieces.
5. Now slice the radishes and finely dice the spring onion, culantro and snow pea sprouts.
6. Pull the alfafa sprouts by hand and then place all the chopped Ingredients: into a large bowl along with the dressing.
7. Serve the salad topped with avocado half. Alternatively, you can also chop the avocado and slowly fold it into the salad.
8. Sprinkle with a little sesame seeds and serve the salad garnished with lemon juice.
9. Nutritional information per (16 oz.) serving: Calories: 206 Fat: 10.26g Carbohydrates: 25.79g Protein: 7.2g

Chapter 7. Snack

Bean Burgers

Preparation time: 20 minutes

Cooking time: 25 minutes

Servings: 8

Ingredients:

- ½ cup walnuts
- 1 carrot, peeled and chopped
- 1 celery stalk, chopped
- 4 scallions, chopped
- 5 garlic cloves, chopped
- 2¼ cups canned black beans, rinsed and drained
- 2½ cups sweet potato, peeled and grated
- ½ teaspoon red pepper flakes, crushed
- ¼ teaspoon cayenne pepper
- Sea salt and freshly ground black pepper, to taste

Directions:

1. Preheat the oven to 400 degrees F. Line a baking sheet with parchment paper.
2. In a food processor, add the walnuts and pulse until finely ground.
3. Add the carrot, celery, scallion, and garlic and pulse until chopped finely.
4. Transfer the vegetable mixture into a large bowl.
5. In the same food processor, add the beans and pulse until chopped.
6. Add 1½ cups of the sweet potato and pulse until a chunky mixture forms.
7. Transfer the bean mixture into the bowl with the vegetable mixture.
8. Stir in remaining sweet potato and spices and mix until well combined.
9. Make 8 equal sized patties from the mixture.
10. Arrange the patties onto the prepared baking sheet in a single layer.
11. Bake for about 25 minutes.
12. Serve hot.

Nutrition: Calories 300 Total Fat 5.5 g Saturated Fat 0.5 g Cholesterol 0 mg Sodium 65 mg Total Carbs 49.8 g Fiber 11.4g Sugar 5.9 g Protein 15.3 g

Grilled Watermelon

Preparation time: 10 minutes

Cooking time: 4 minutes

Servings: 4

Ingredients:

- 1 watermelon, peeled and cut into 1-inch thick wedges
- 1 garlic clove, minced finely
- 2 tablespoons fresh lime juice
- Pinch of cayenne pepper
- Pinch of sea salt

Directions:

1. Preheat the grill to high heat. Grease the grill grate.
2. Grill the watermelon pieces for about 2 minutes on both sides.
3. Meanwhile, in a small bowl mix together the remaining Ingredients:.
4. Drizzle the watermelon slices with the lemon mixture and serve.

Nutrition: Calories 11 Total Fat 0.1 g Saturated Fat 0 g Cholesterol 0 mg Sodium 59 mg Total Carbs 2.6 g Fiber 0.2 g Sugar 1.9 g Protein 0.2 g

---

Mango Salsa

Preparation time: 15 minutes

Servings: 6

Ingredients:

- 1 avocado, peeled, pitted, and cut into cubes
- 2 tablespoons fresh lime juice
- 1 mango, peeled, pitted, and cubed
- 1 cup cherry tomatoes, halved
- 1 jalapeño pepper, seeded and chopped
- 1 tablespoon fresh cilantro, chopped
- Sea salt, to taste

Directions:

1. In a large bowl, add the avocado and lime juice and mix well.
2. Add the remaining Ingredients: and stir to combine.
3. Serve immediately.

Nutrition: Calories 108 Total Fat 6.8 g Saturated Fat 1.4 g Cholesterol 0 mg Sodium 43 mg Total Carbs 12.6 g Fiber 3.6 g Sugar 8.7 g Protein 1.4 g

Avocado Gazpacho

Preparation time: 15 minutes

Servings: 6

Ingredients:

- 3 large avocados, peeled, pitted, and chopped
- 1/3 cup fresh cilantro leaves
- 3 cups homemade vegetable broth
- 2 tablespoons fresh lemon juice
- 1 teaspoon ground cumin
- ¼ teaspoon cayenne pepper
- Sea salt, to taste

Directions:

1. Add all the Ingredients: in a high-speed blender and pulse until smooth.
2. Transfer the soup into a large bowl.
3. Cover the bowl and refrigerate to chill for at least 2-3 hours before serving.

Nutrition: Calories 227 Total Fat 20.4 g Saturated Fat 4.4 g Cholesterol 0 mg Sodium 429 mg Total Carbs 9.4 g Fiber 6.8 g Sugar 1 g Protein 4.5 g

---

Roasted Chickpeas

Preparation time: 10 minutes

Cooking time: 45 minutes

Servings: 12

Ingredients:

- 4 cups cooked chickpeas
- 2 garlic cloves, minced
- ½ teaspoon dried oregano, crushed
- ½ teaspoon smoked paprika
- ¼ teaspoon ground cumin
- Sea salt, to taste
- 1 tablespoon olive oil

Directions:

1. Preheat the oven to 400 degrees F. Grease a large baking sheet.
2. Place chickpeas onto the prepared baking sheet in a single layer.
3. Roast for about 30 minutes, stirring the chickpeas every 10 minutes.
4. Meanwhile, in a small mixing bowl, mix together garlic, thyme, and spices.
5. Remove the baking sheet from the oven.
6. Pour the garlic mixture and oil over the chickpeas and toss to coat well.
7. Roast for about 10-15 minutes more.

8. Now, turn the oven off but leave the baking sheet inside for about 10 minutes before serving.

Nutrition: Calories 92 Total Fat 1.9 g Saturated Fat 0.2 g Cholesterol 0 mg Sodium 166 mg Total Carbs 15 g Fiber 0.1 g Sugar 4 g Protein 4.1 g

---

Banana Chips

Preparation time: 10 minutes

Cooking time: 1 hour 10 minutes

Servings: 4

Ingredients:

- 2 large bananas, peeled and cut into ¼-inch thick slices

Directions:

1. Prepare the oven to 250 degrees F. Line a large baking sheet with baking paper.
2. Place the banana slices onto the prepared baking sheet in a single layer.
3. Bake for about 1 hour.

Nutrition: Calories 61 Total Fat 0.2 g Saturated Fat 0.1 g Cholesterol 0 mg Sodium 1 mg Total Carbs 15.5 g Fiber 1.8 g Sugar 8.3 g Protein 0.7 g

---

Roasted Cashews

Preparation time: 10 minutes

Cooking time: 10 minutes

Servings: 12

Ingredients:

- 2 cups raw cashews
- ½ teaspoon ground cumin
- ¼ teaspoon cayenne pepper
- Pinch of salt
- 1 tablespoon fresh lemon juice

Directions:

1. Preheat the oven to 400 degrees F. Line a large roasting pan with a piece of foil.
2. In a large bowl, add the cashews and spices and toss to coat well.
3. Transfer the cashews to the prepared roasting pan.
4. Roast for about 8-10 minutes.

5. Drizzle with lemon juice and serve.

Nutrition: Calories 132 Total Fat 10.6 g Saturated Fat 2.1 g Cholesterol 0 mg Sodium 16 mg Total Carbs 7.6 g Fiber 0.7 g Sugar 1.2 g Protein 3.5 g

---

Dried Orange Slices

Preparation time: 10 minutes

Cooking time: 10 hours Total time: 10 hours 10 minutes

Servings: 15

Ingredients:

- 4 seedless navel oranges, cut into thin slices (do NOT peel oranges)

Directions:

1. Set the dehydrator to 135 degrees F.
2. Arrange the orange slices onto the dehydrator sheets.
3. Dehydrate for about 10 hours.

Nutrition: Calories 23 Total Fat 0.1 g Saturated Fat 0 g Cholesterol 0 mg Sodium 0 mg Total Carbs 5.8 g Fiber 3.5 g Sugar 4.6 g Protein 0.5 g

---

Chickpea Hummus

Preparation time: 10 minutes

Servings: 12

Ingredients:

- 2 (15-ounce) cans chickpeas, rinsed and drained
- ½ cup tahini
- 1 garlic clove, chopped
- 2 tablespoons fresh lemon juice
- Sea salt, to taste
- Filtered water, as needed
- 1 tablespoon olive oil plus more for drizzling
- Pinch of cayenne pepper

Directions:

1. In a blender, add all the Ingredients: and pulse until smooth.
2. Transfer the hummus into a large bowl and drizzle with oil.
3. Sprinkle with cayenne pepper and serve immediately.

Nutrition: Calories 129 Total Fat 7.4 g Saturated Fat 0.9 g Cholesterol 0 mg Sodium 19521 mg Total Carbs 12.2 g Fiber 3.3 g Sugar 1.2 g Protein 4.7 g

---

Baked Avocado Fries

Prep time: 7 minutes, Cook time: 17 minutes

Serves 4

Ingredients:

- ½ cup almond flour
- ½ teaspoon ground paprika, plus more for sprinkling
- 2 tablespoons nutritional yeast
- ½ teaspoon garlic powder
- 2 avocados, slightly underripe
- ½ cup almond milk
- ½ teaspoon sea salt

Directions:

1. Preheat the oven to 420°F.
2. In a small bowl, stir together the almond flour, nutritional yeast, garlic powder, paprika, and salt until well combined.
3. Halve and pit the avocados, and quarter each half from pole to pole. Peel off the skin.
4. Add the almond milk to another small bowl.
5. Line a baking sheet with parchment paper.
6. Dip an avocado slice into first the milk and then the coating mixture, gently tossing it to make sure it is completely covered, and place on the prepared baking sheet. Repeat with the remaining avocado slices.
7. Bake for 15 to 17 minutes, taking care not to overcook or burn them.
8. Remove from oven, sprinkle with additional paprika, and serve immediately.

Dried Cinnamon Apples

Prep time: 3 minutes, Cook time: 3 hours

Serves 1

Ingredients:

- 2 apples, sliced
- 1 teaspoon ground cinnamon
- 1 teaspoon olive oil

Directions:

1. Spread all the apple slices on a baking sheet.

2. Toss the slices with cinnamon and olive oil.
3. Bake for 3 hours at 200 degrees F.
4. Serve and enjoy!

Salsa Guacamole

Prep time: 5 minutes

Serves 1

Ingredients:

- ½ cup salsa,
- 2 smashed avocados,
- 2 tablespoons chopped cilantro
- Salt, to taste

Directions:

1. Mix all the Ingredients: in a bowl.
2. Serve and enjoy!

Apple Chips

Prep time: 3 minutes, Cook time: 40 minutes

Serves 2

Ingredients:

- 2 apples, cored and sliced thinly
- 2 tsps. white sugar
- ½ tsps. ground cinnamon

Directions:

1. Preheat oven to 225 degrees F.
2. Put the apple slices on a baking sheet.
3. Drizzle cinnamon and sugar.
4. Bake for 40 minutes and then serve.

Quick Alka-Goulash

Prep time: 10 minutes, Cook time: 15 minutes

Serves 4

Ingredients:

- 1 onion, finely chopped
- 1 clove of garlic, crushed
- 2 carrots, diced
- 3 zucchinis, diced
- 2 tbsp. olive oil
- 1 tbsp. paprika
- ¼ tsp. ground nutmeg
- 1 tbsp. fresh parsley, chopped
- 1 tbsp. tomato purée
- 2 cups of tomatoes, peeled
- 2 cups cooked red kidney beans, drained and rinsed
- ½ cup tomato juice
- Salt and black pepper to taste

Directions:

1. Sauté the onion, garlic, carrot and zucchini in olive oil over medium heat for 5 minutes until softened.
2. Stir in the paprika, nutmeg, parsley and tomato puree.
3. Add the tomatoes, red kidney beans and tomato juice, and stir.
4. Simmer for 10 minutes until warmed through.
5. Serve immediately. Enjoy!

Eggplant "Caviar"

Known as "Poor Man's Caviar," this is an absolutely delicious eggplant purée that you'll want to eat all day long! Eggplant is a great source of copper, vitamin B1 and fiber, and any dish that uses this deep purple beauty is worthy of including on any menu.

Servings: 2-4

Ingredients:

- 2 medium eggplants
- 2 tbsps. olive oil
- 1 onion, finely chopped
- 1 green bell pepper, deseeded and finely chopped
- 2 tbsps. tomato purée
- 4 tbsps. water
- 2 tbsps. lemon juice
- Salt and black pepper to taste
- Gluten-free bread or wrap of your choice

Instructions:

1. Pierce the eggplants several times with a sharp knife. Boil or steam them until soft. Allow them to cool.
2. Remove the stems and scoop the flesh out of the eggplants. Finely chop the soft flesh.
3. Add the olive oil to a large frying pan over a medium heat. Sauté the onion and green bell pepper until the onion is translucent.
4. Add the eggplant, tomato purée, water, salt and black pepper to the pan.
5. Reduce the heat and cook over the lowest possible heat. Stir frequently for 20-30 minutes, at which point the mixture will start to thicken.
6. Place the mixture in a bowl and stir in the lemon juice.
7. Allow the mixture to cool and place it in the fridge.
8. Serve chilled with a slice of gluten-free bread, wrap or chopped veggies (e.g. carrots or cucumbers).

Spicy Nut Mix

Owing to the fact that most fruits and vegetables are low in both fat and protein, it often falls upon nuts and seeds to pick up the shortfall in a vegan-style diets. As used in this wonderful mix, hazelnuts are also particularly rich in vitamin E and manganese which are great for your skin and overall health and wellbeing.

Serves: 4

Ingredients:

- 1/3 cup sesame seeds
- 1/2 cup hazelnuts, blanched
- 3 tbsp. coriander seeds
- 2 tbsp. cumin seeds
- Warm gluten-free tortilla wraps of your choice, sliced into strips or chopped veggies
- Olive oil
- 1/2 tsp. salt
- Black pepper to taste

Instructions

1. Dry fry the sesame seeds in a large pan over a medium heat, until they are golden. Remove from the heat and allow to cool in a bowl.
2. Toast the hazelnuts in the same pan until they are shining are starting to turn golden. Add to the sesame seeds and allow to cool.
3. Dry fry the coriander and cumin seeds until fragrant but be sure not to allow them to burn. Add them to the bowl of hazelnuts and sesame seeds and allow to cool.

4. Now put the mixture into a food processor and add salt and black pepper to taste. Process the mixture until it gains the consistency of a coarse, dry powder.
5. Serve with gluten-free tortillas wraps or veggies next to a bowl of olive oil. To consume, dip the bread or raw veggies, in the oil and then in the spicy nut mixture.

Garlic Mushrooms

Garlic is miraculous and a great source of all kinds of minerals and antioxidants. Combined with the protein-packed punch from a healthy serving of mushrooms, this dish is bound to give your mealtimes a boost. By the way, mushrooms are not really alkaline and should only be eaten sparingly as your 20-30%, but as we have already concluded, the alkaline diet is not only about eating 100% alkaline foods.

Serves: 4

Ingredients:

- 2 tbsp. olive oil
- 2 cloves of garlic, crushed
- 1/4 tsp dried thyme
- 1/4 tsp dried parsley
- 1/4 tsp dried sage
- 2 cups mushrooms, chopped into quarters
- Chopped raw veggies of your choice (e.g. cucumbers, carrots, bell peppers)
- 2 tbsp. chives, chopped
- Salt and black pepper to taste

Instructions:

1. Sauté the garlic in olive oil until it softens and begins to brown.
2. Add the dried herbs and mushrooms and season with salt and black pepper to taste. Sauté this mixture over a low heat for around 10 minutes, until the mushrooms are soft.
3. Serve the mushrooms alongside raw veggies. Garnish with the chopped chives.
4. Enjoy!

Hummus

Hummus is a classic dip from the Middle East, which incorporates some of the tastiest **Ingredients:** in the region. Chickpeas provide you with a valuable source of carbohydrates and protein, while the tahini and olive oil give you a good source of healthy plant fats. It's simply delicious as a start or snack!

Ingredients:

- 1 cup cooked chickpeas, broth reserved
- 4 tbsp. light tahini
- Juice of 2 lemons
- 6 tbsp. olive oil
- 4 cloves of garlic, crushed
- Salt to taste

Instructions:

1. Blend the chickpeas with 1/8 cup of broth reserved from the cooking process.
2. Add the lemon juice, garlic, tahini and half of the olive oil.
3. Blend this mixture until smooth.
4. Leave to stand for around an hour before serving.
5. To serve, drizzle the remaining olive oil over each individual portion. Serve alongside some raw veggies.

Zucchini Vegan Paleo Hummus

This is a great option for those who don't like legumes. All you need to do is to replace chickpeas with zucchini. I also like to add some cilantro. Zucchini can be raw or slightly cooked, it's up to you. You may even stir-fry it in coconut oil for more amazing flavour.

Ingredients:

- 1 cup zucchini slices
- 4 tbsps. light tahini
- Juice of 2 lemons
- 6 tbsps. olive oil
- 4 cloves of garlic, crushed
- Himalayan salt to taste

Instructions:

1. Combine zucchini, lemon juice, garlic, tahini and half of the olive oil in a blender.
2. Blend this mixture until smooth.
3. Leave to stand for around an hour before serving.
4. To serve, drizzle the remaining olive oil over each individual portion. Serve alongside some raw veggies or sprouted bread.

German-style Sweet Potato Salad

This healthy, alkaline version of traditional potato salad is packed with herbs, giving you a delicious source of minerals like iron and magnesium. The potatoes will give you a nice long-lasting energy boost, too!

Servings: 2-4

Ingredients:

- 2 cups sweet potatoes, chopped
- 1 cup baby spinach
- 1 cup cherry tomatoes
- 1 red bell pepper
- 4 tbsps. olive oil
- 4 scallions, trimmed and finely chopped
- 1 clove of garlic, crushed or minced
- 2 tbsps. fresh dill, finely chopped
- 2 tbsps. fresh parsley, chopped
- Salt and black pepper to taste

Instructions:

1. Clean and peel the potatoes. Boil them in a saucepan until just tender. The time required will vary depending on their size.
2. Meanwhile, sauté the garlic and scallions in a frying pan over a medium heat for 2-3 minutes, until slightly soft.
3. Add the dill and sauté for around 1 minute.
4. Remove from the heat and season to taste with the salt and black pepper.
5. Drain the potatoes once cooked, and pour the herb dressing over the top while they are hot.
6. Allow to cool and then add the rest of the Ingredients: and garnish with the parsley. Serve chilled!

Quinoa Salad

This is another super quick-prep dish. Just remember to cook your quinoa in batches to be sure you always have some ready to grab from your fridge. This meal also makes an excellent take away lunch.

Serves: 2

Ingredients:

- 1 cup quinoa, cooked
- 1 garlic clove, minced
- 1 cucumber, chopped
- 1 cup fresh arugula leaves
- 1 red bell pepper, chopped

- 1 big avocado, peeled, pitted and diced
- 2 tablespoons chia seeds (optional)
- 2 tablespoons olive oil
- 2 tablespoons coconut milk (think)
- Himalayan salt and black pepper to taste
- Juice of 1 lime or lemon

Instructions:

1. Simply combine all the Ingredients: in a big salad bowl.
2. Toss well and sprinkle over some olive oil, coconut milk and lemon juice.
3. Enjoy!

Tasty Quinoa Coconut Salad

In case you find quinoa a bit dull, try this recipe. It will give you inspiration as for how you can experiment with all kinds of exotic flavours on the alkaline diet and transform different foods to enjoy more variety.

Serves: 2

Ingredients:

- 2 cups quinoa, cooked
- 3 tablespoons coconut oil
- 1 garlic clove, minced
- 1 teaspoon curry powder
- 1 teaspoon cilantro powder
- ½ teaspoon garlic powder
- 1 cup radish
- 1/2 cup arugula leaves
- 2 horse radishes, sliced super thin or spiralized
- ¼ cup raisins
- Himalayan salt to taste
- 1 lime

Instructions:

1. Heat some coconut oil in a pan (low or medium, heat).
2. Add garlic and sauté for a couple of minutes.
3. Then add quinoa, curry powder and garlic powder.
4. Keep stirring on low heat so that quinoa takes a nice exotic flavour.
5. Add a pinch of Himalayan salt to taste. You can also add some coconut milk.
6. Turn off the heat and let quinoa cool down.
7. In the meantime, combine the remaining Ingredients: in a salad bowl.
8. Add quinoa, toss well, and sprinkle over some lime juice.
9. Serve chilled.
10. Enjoy!

Mayo Alkaline Salad

If you fear eating salads because you fear you will not feel full for too long, try this one. It offers a perfect combination of refreshment that you typically get after eating a salad, but at the same time, it will keep your belly full. This salad leaves plenty of room for personalization in case you want to add other Ingredients:. Great all year long!

Serves: 4

Ingredients:

- 2 cups sweet potato, boiled, sliced, chilled
- 1 cup soy sprouts (I am not talking about soy, but soy sprouts...)
- 2 red bell peppers, chopped
- 1 onion, chopped
- 1 cup arugula leaves

- ¼ cup almond, crushed
- ½ cup vegan mayonnaise
- Juice of 1 lime
- 2 tablespoons olive oil
- Himalayan salt and black pepper to taste

Instructions:

1. Combine all the Ingredients: in a big salad bowl.
2. Add vegan mayo, olive oil, lemon juice, black pepper and salt.
3. Mix well. Cool down in a refrigerator for a couple of hours.
4. Serve chilled and enjoy!

Black-eyed Peas and Orange Salad

It's becoming increasingly popular to include fruit as part of an otherwise savoury salad. This is great for us "alkalarians" as it adds another nutritional dimension to the dish. Oranges, even though not super alkalizing, are well known for being high in vitamin C and make a great accompaniment to the protein-rich black-eyed peas. Balanced diet is the key to success. We should not fear fruit.

Servings: 4

Ingredients:

- 1 cup black-eyed peas, soaked
- 1 bay leaf
- A slice of onion
- Zest and juice of 1 orange
- 5 tbsp. olive oil

- 6 large olives, pitted and chopped
- 4 scallions, trimmed and chopped
- 2 tbsp. fresh parsley, chopped
- 2 tbsp. fresh basil, chopped
- 4 whole oranges

- 1 large handful of watercress

Instructions

1. Put the black-eyes peas, bay leaf and onion slice in a saucepan filled with enough water to cover them by 1 inch.
2. Boil at a high heat for 10 minutes, then reduce to a simmer and cook for 60 minutes, until the black-eyed peas are soft.
3. Whisk the olive oil, orange rind and juice in a bowl.
4. Add the olives, scallions and herbs, then mix.
5. Drain the black-eyed peas and add them to the mixture.
6. Season to taste and ensure that the black-eyed peas are well-coated by the mixture.
7. Serve the mixture on individual plates, and add some orange segments and a pile of watercress to each.

Quick Alka-Goulash

Inspired the Hungarian classic of the same name, this speedy version of Goulash is a flavor explosion! The generous portion of cooked tomatoes included mean that you'll be getting plenty of antioxidants, lycopene in particular.

Servings: 4

Ingredients:

- 1 onion, finely chopped
- 1 clove of garlic, crushed
- 2 carrots, diced
- 3 zucchini, diced
- 2 tbsp. olive oil
- 1 tbsp. paprika
- 1/4 tsp. ground nutmeg
- 1 tbsp. fresh parsley, chopped
- 1 tbsp. tomato purée
- 2 cups of tomatoes, peeled
- 2 cups cooked red kidney beans, drained and rinsed
- 1/2 cup tomato juice
- Salt and black pepper to taste

Instructions

1. Sauté the onion, garlic, carrot and zucchini in olive oil over a medium heat for 5 minutes, until softened.
2. Stir in the paprika, nutmeg, parsley and tomato puree.
3. Add the tomatoes, red kidney beans and tomato juice, and stir.
4. Simmer for 10 minutes until warmed through.
5. Serve immediately. Enjoy!

Pea Risotto

One of the great classics of rice-based cuisine, risotto is often made with the addition of butter or some kind of meat or poultry which are acid-forming. Fortunately, this simply doesn't have to be the case. A perfectly delicious risotto can be made without any of these things in a more alkaline friendly and vegan way.

Servings: 4

Ingredients:

- 1 vegetable broth cube
- 2 tbsp. olive oil
- 1 onion, finely chopped
- 3 cloves of garlic, finely chopped
- 1 cup basmati rice
- 1 cup frozen peas
- 1 cup fresh baby spinach leaves
- 1 lemon, grated and juiced
- Salt and black pepper to taste
- 3 cups water

Instructions

1. Crumble the vegetable broth cube into 3 cups of boiling water. Allow it to dissolve and then reduce the heat.
2. Defrost the peas in warm water, drain and set aside for later.
3. Season the onion with salt and black pepper to taste, and then sauté it in olive oil at a medium heat for around 5 minutes, until softened.
4. Add the garlic to the frying pan and sauté for a few minutes, ensuring that it doesn't burn.
5. Add the rice to the frying pan and mix well. Ladle in some vegetable broth so that the rice is just covered.
6. Simmer over medium heat while constantly stirring for a few minutes, until the liquid has been almost completely absorbed.
7. Add the rest of the broth a ladleful at a time, stirring constantly until each batch of broth has been absorbed.
8. After each ladleful has been absorbed and the rice is fully cooked, add the defrosted peas, baby spinach leaves and lemon juice.
9. Stir until the baby spinach leaves have wilted and then serve while hot.
10. Enjoy!

Satisfying Alka-Lunch Smoothie

I know what you're thinking. Is Marta putting her alkaline breakfast recipes into a lunch cookbook? Well, I can understand your confusion and usually I don't have smoothies for lunch, however I think there is nothing wrong with that. Especially if you are pressed for time. This is what I do whenever I am in rush; I just make myself a satisfying, nutritious smoothie that keeps me full till my mid-afternoon snack or sometimes even until dinner!

Servings: 1-2

Ingredients:

- 1 big avocado
- 1.5 cup coconut milk or almond milk
- 2 tablespoons fresh cilantro leaves
- 2 tablespoons coconut oil
- 1 lemon, juiced
- 4 tablespoons of chia seeds
- Himalayan salt to taste

Instructions:

1. Simply blend all the Ingredients: except seeds and oil.
2. Stir well, add chia seeds and taste with Himalayan salt.
3. Enjoy!

Alkaline Pizza Bread

This is one recipe that is rich in fiber, calcium, iron, omega-3, and vitamins. Flax seeds are very nutritional, and their presence alone makes each recipe worthwhile. I've been exploring to see the impact they have on human health and I was so impressed to find out that they are not only anti-carcinogenic, they also help reduce blood sugar, control cholesterol, and even aid weight control.

Sunflower seed, on the other hand, supports skin health, promotes restful sleep, fights hypertension and aids hair growth.

The pizza bread is a very healthy snack that comes highly recommended.

Servings: One (1)

Ingredients:

- Flax seeds, 100g
- Sunflower seeds, 200g
- Pepper, a pinch
- Sundried tomatoes, 50g
- Organic or sea salt, a pinch
- Extra virgin olive oil (cold pressed), 4 teaspoons
- Optional: Fresh wild garlic

Directions:

1. Note: You have to soak the sunflower seeds for at least four hours.
2. Blend the flax seeds in a blender until it turns to powder.
3. Once the sunflower seeds have lasted up to four hours, put them in a blender and blend for some seconds.
4. Now add all the Ingredients: in a mixing bowl.
5. With your hands, form a dough until you reach a right consistency.
6. The idea is to form a couple of pizza crusts/bread.
7. Put them in a dehydrator or oven and dehydrate for up to twelve hours.
8. Serve.

Alkaline Filled Avocados

Scientifically, avocados are known to kill cancer cells, lower cholesterol levels in the blood and also regulate blood pressure. So whenever you see avocado in any meal, you should at least reserve some level of excitement because it means that you're definitely enriching your body to a reasonable extent.

Moreover, some nutrients in this healthy alkaline avocado snack include potassium and oleic acid, which play some proactive roles in the body.

Basil, an ingredient in this recipe contains compounds that serve as immune boosters, pain reducers, cancer fighters, and antioxidants.

The Alkaline filled Avocado is a recipe that will leave you fulfilled, contented and happy.

Servings: one (1)

Ingredients:

- Oregano, 1 teaspoon
- Ripe avocado, 1
- Lime juice (fresh), 1 teaspoon
- Fresh basil, 1 teaspoon
- Minced onions, 1 teaspoon
- Tomato, ½
- Extra virgin oil (Cold pressed), 4 teaspoons
- Pepper and sea salt

Directions:

1. Slice avocado into two equal halves and remove the seed.
2. Use salt and pepper to season both halves.
3. Mix the olive oil, minced onion, lime juice, and chopped tomato, and place in the avocado pit holes.
4. Spray oregano and basil on top and serve.

Alkalized Potato Salad

Red potatoes are gluten-free foods that help boost the immune system, regulate blood pressure, and reduce stress levels. They are delicious energy giving foods that complement a lot of other condiments in meals. So when you make a meal with potatoes and dill, you'll end up with a very healthy blend e.g., dill helps reduce menstrual cramps, fights depression and lowers cholesterol, as well as aids digestion.

The alkalized potato salad is a unique delicacy.

Servings: Four (4)

Ingredients:

- Cauliflower, 1 cup
- Dill, 2 tablespoons
- Vegenaise, 1 teaspoon
- Red onion, 1
- English cucumber (small), 1
- Broccoli, 2 cups
- Green/ red pepper (small), 1
- Red potatoes, 600g
- Juice of 1 lemon
- Sea salt
- Olive oil (Cold pressed), 3 tablespoons

Directions:

1. Steam cauliflower and broccoli for some minutes and make sure they are crunchy.
2. Also, steam potatoes until they are mildly soft and allow them to cool.
3. Once they are cool, slice the potatoes but do not remove the skin and dump in a big bowl.
4. Next, add the chopped cucumber, cauliflower, pepper, broccoli, along with the dill, the finely chopped onion, and the salt.
5. Mix properly and set aside.
6. Get a small bowl and mix the veganaise, olive oil, and lemon juice until you get a smooth dressing.
7. Mix it in the potato salad and toss mildly.
8. You can serve immediately but it is better to put it aside for some hours (because it tastes better that way).
9. You are free to add more seasonings to your taste.

Almonds With Stir-Fried Greens

This is another highly rated snack that is so soothing to the taste bud. The stir greens with almonds come fully loaded with beans, broccoli, lemon juice, and cauliflowers, etc. It is nutrient rich, easy to fix and delicious.

Another aspect to it is the fact that it is 100% fresh, health and alkaline!

Yummy!

Servings: Four (4)

Ingredients:

- Young beans, 150g
- Flower of broccoli, 4
- Oregano and cumin, ½ teaspoon
- Lemon juice (fresh), 3 tablespoons
- Garlic clove (finely chopped), 1
- Cauliflower, 1 cup
- Olive oil (cold pressed), 4 tablespoons
- Pepper and salt to taste
- Some soaked almonds (sliced), for garnishing
- Yellow onion, 1

Directions:

1. Add broccoli, beans, and other vegetables in a large pan and fry until beans and broccoli turns dark green.
2. Make sure the vegetables are crunchy too.
3. Now add chopped garlic and onion, stir fry and mix for some few minutes.
4. Next, put together the dressing.
5. Get a small bowl, add lemon juice, oregano, cumin, and oil, and mix properly.
6. Add some vegetables, mix slowly, and taste with pepper and salt.
7. Lastly, use the sliced almonds to garnish it.
8. Serve.

Alkaline Sweet Potato Mash

Sweet potatoes are a natural antioxidant rich in vitamins C and A, and low in calories. While fresh coconut milk is rich in Lauric Acids (which are renowned for their antiviral, antimicrobial and anticarcinogenic abilities).

Sweet potatoes are perfect for diabetic patients because they help stabilize blood sugar, as well as reduce blood.

So when you opt for this meal, you are actually giving yourself an all-around treat (easy to make, delicious and beneficial to your health).

Servings: three (3) – Four (4)

Ingredients:

- Sea salt, 1 tablespoon
- Curry powder, ½ tablespoon
- Sweet potatoes (large), 6
- Coconut milk (fresh), 1 ½ - 2 cups
- Extra virgin oil (cold pressed), 1 tablespoon
- Pepper, 1 pinch

Directions:

1. First, get a large cooking bowl.
2. Wash and chop the sweet potatoes and add in the cooking bowl and cook for around twenty minutes.
3. Next, take off the sweet potatoes and mash to your desired consistency.
4. Finally, all you have to do is to add the remaining Ingredients: and serve.

Mediterranean Bell Peppers

Bell peppers are low-calorie alkaline foods that are enriched with Vitamin B6, Vitamin C, folic acid, and thiamine and beta carotene.

They are known to prevent certain forms of cancer, reduce strokes and heart attacks, as well as strengthen the immune system.

Apart from the health mentioned above benefits, they also taste outstanding when used in cooking.

Servings: Two (2)

Ingredients:

- Oregano, 1 teaspoon
- Garlic cloves (crushed), 2
- Fresh parsley (chopped), 2 tablespoons
- Vegetable stock (yeast free), 1 cup
- Herbs of the province, 1 teaspoon
- Red bell pepper (sliced) 2 + yellow bell pepper (sliced) 2
- Red onions (thinly sliced), 2 medium sized
- Extra virgin oil (cold pressed), 2 tablespoons
- Salt and pepper to taste

Directions:

1. Heat up olive oil in a pan over medium heat, add bell pepper and onions, and stir.
2. Add the garlic and stir.

3. Next, add the vegetable stock and season with parsley and herbs, as well as pepper and salt to taste.
4. Cover the pan and let it cook for fourteen to fifteen minutes.
5. Serve.

Tomato-Avocado-Salsa with Potatoes

This delicious alkaline menu is rich in potassium, fiber, iron, and calcium and is ideal when there are visitors around.

In as much as it is healthy and alkaline, it's still versatile in the sense that healthy and non–healthy eaters would enjoy it all the same.

Servings: Two (2) – Three (3)

Ingredients:

- Red onion (small), 1
- Tomatoes (average size), 2
- ½ - 1 lemon (juiced)
- Chives (fresh and chopped), 1 teaspoon
- Parsley (fresh and chopped), 1 teaspoon
- Cayenne pepper, ½ teaspoon
- Avocados (ripe), 2
- Waxy potatoes (average size), 6
- Saltwater
- Pepper and salt

Directions:

1. Get a cooking pan and cook the potatoes in salt water, (cook potatoes with the skin intact).
2. Next, peel the avocado, throw in a bowl and mash with a fork.
3. Now, dice the onion and tomatoes, add them in the bowl along with the parsley, chives, and cayenne.
4. Mix it properly and season with pepper, lemon juice, and salt.
5. Serve along with the potatoes.

Alkaline Green beans & Coconut

Green beans are packed with fiber which helps control high blood pressure. They are also enriched with Potassium, Manganese, Vitamins A, C, and K, and are extremely low in calories.

Coconut milk is known to lower cholesterols level and also contain Lauric acid which makes it antiviral, anti-bacterial, anti-carcinogenic and anti-microbial.

Garlic is rich in selenium, fiber, calcium, phosphorus, iron, and copper. It is known to help protect heart health and reduce blood pressure.

Green beans help reduce colon cancer risks, boost immunity; treat gastrointestinal issues and boosts eyesight.

This recipe is healthy and nutritious, try it out.

Servings: Four (4)

Ingredients:

- Ground cumin, ½ teaspoon
- Red chili (chopped), 1-2
- Coconut milk (fresh), 3 tablespoons
- Dried flaked coconut, 1tablespoon
- Garlic (chopped), 2 cloves
- Cayenne pepper, 1 pinch
- Sea salt, 1 pinch
- Extra virgin oil (cold pressed), 3 tablespoons
- Fresh herbs of your choice, 1 teaspoon
- One (1) Pound green (string) beans, cut in 1-inch pieces
- Fresh ginger (chopped), ½ teaspoon

Directions:

1. Heat oil in a frying pan and add the beans, cumin, garlic, ginger, and chill, and stir-fry for about six minutes.
2. Add the coconut flakes and oil and stir-fry until the milk is wholly vaporized (this might take three to four minutes).
3. Season with pepper, salt, and herbs to taste.
4. Serve.

Alkalized Vegetable Lasagna

Avocados, as we already know, are anti-carcinogenic (they fight against certain forms of cancer, especially breast and prostate cancer).

Minerals such as Potassium and Oleic acid present in avocados help regulate blood pressure, as well as lower blood cholesterol, respectively.

Garlic contains Vitamins B1, B6, C, Selenium, Manganese, Fiber, Calcium, Copper, Phosphorus, and Iron. Garlic contains active compounds that reduce blood pressure and lower risks of heart disease.

Radish helps supply oxygen to the blood, controls blood pressure, helps reduce cardiovascular diseases, improves immunity and promotes hydration.

Leeks fight anemia, improves eyesight, strengthens the bones and fights certain forms of cancer risks.

Arugula is an aphrodisiac. It aids weight loss, protects the aging brain from cognitive decline, detoxifies the body, and hydrates the body.

Enjoy this nutrient-packed recipe.

Servings: one (1)

Ingredients:

- Parsley root, 1
- Leek (small), 1
- Radish (small), 1
- Corn salad, 1
- Tomatoes (big), 3
- Garlic, 1 clove
- Avocados (soft), 2
- Lemon (juiced), 1-2
- Arugula, 1
- Parsley (few)
- Red bell pepper, 1

Directions:

1. Get a blender and add the following; the lemon juice, garlic clove, and avocados.
2. Cut the bell pepper into thin strips, cut the leek into fine rings, and finely grate the parsley root and the radish. When you are done, mix it with the avocado cream.
3. Let's start with the first layer of the lasagna.
4. Deposit the corn salad in a casserole, add the avocado spread well.
5. For the second layer, add sliced tomatoes.
6. Lastly, add the arugula and the parsley for the final layer.
7. Serve.

Aloo Gobi

This Mediterranean recipe comes loaded with taste, flavor, and nutrients. It is delicious, nutrient-rich and easy to prepare.

As per its health benefits, cauliflower is high in fiber and an antioxidant. It fights inflammation, promotes heart health, reduces certain cancer risks, improves digestion and detoxification. Cauliflower is also an anti-aging agent; it boosts the immune system, as well as boosts brain health.

Ginger combats morning sickness, relieves muscle pain, relieves Osteoarthritis, lowers blood sugar and improves heart health. It also reduces cholesterol levels and prevents certain types of cancer.

Mint contains fiber, Vitamin A, Manganese, Iron and Folate. It helps improve irritable bowel syndrome, relieves indigestion, improves brain function, decreases breastfeeding pain and helps reduce bad breath.

Turmeric is anti-inflammatory; it promotes heart health and contains anti-carcinogenic properties.

Garlic combats common cold, improves cholesterol levels, reduces blood pressure and contains compounds that help prevent Alzheimer's disease.

Tomatoes are antioxidants and are rich in vitamins and minerals. They contain compounds that aid digestion, lower hypertension, improve eyesight, manage diabetes and prevent gallstones.

Coriander reduces skin inflammation, relieves skin disorders, lowers cholesterol levels and treats diarrhea. It also regulates blood pressure, heals mouth ulcers, and conjunctivitis.

Potatoes contain fat, protein, carbs, and fiber, Vitamins C, B6, Potassium, Manganese, and Magnesium. They help control blood sugar, improve digestive health, and are antioxidants.

Servings: 1 bowl

Ingredients:

- Cauliflower, 750g
- Fresh ginger, 20g
- Large onions, 2
- Mint, 1/3 cup
- Turmeric, 2 teaspoons
- Diced tomatoes, 400g
- Fresh garlic, 2 cloves
- Cayenne pepper, 2 teaspoons
- Cilantro/coriander leaves, 1/3 cup
- Large potatoes, 4
- Garam masala, 2 teaspoons
- Green chili, 4
- Water, 3 cups
- Extra virgin oil (cold pressed), 125 ml
- Salt to taste

Directions:

1. Blend chili, garlic, and ginger.
2. Sauté oil in a wok for three minutes and add onion until it turns gold.
3. Add the ground paste and stir fry for a few seconds, then add; garam masala, chili, turmeric, tomatoes and salt.
4. Cook for about five minutes and add all other Ingredients:.
5. Stir for three minutes and add water.
6. Cook until the sauce is thick.
7. Serve with Basmati rice or as a side dish.

Chapter 8. Smoothies, Teas, and Juices

Blueberry Smoothie

Preparation time: 10 minutes

Servings: 2

Ingredients:

- 2 cups frozen blueberries
- 1 small banana
- 1½ cups unsweetened almond milk
- ¼ cup ice cubes

Directions:

1. Place all the Ingredients: in a high-speed blender and pulse until creamy.
2. Pour the smoothie into two glasses and serve immediately.

Nutrition: Calories 158 Total Fat 3.3 g Saturated Fat 0.3 g Cholesterol 0 mg Sodium 137 mg Total Carbs 34 g Fiber 5.6 g Sugar 20.6 g Protein 2.4 g

---

Raspberry & Tofu Smoothie

Preparation time: 10 minutes

Servings: 2

Ingredients:

- 1½ cups fresh raspberries
- 6 ounces firm silken tofu, pressed and drained
- 4-5 drops liquid stevia
- 1 cup coconut cream
- ¼ cup ice, crushed

Directions:

1. Place all the Ingredients: in a high-speed blender and pulse until creamy.
2. Pour the smoothie into two glasses and serve immediately.

Nutrition: Calories 377 Total Fat 31.5 g Saturated Fat 25.7 g Cholesterol 0 mg Sodium 50 mg Total Carbs 19.7 g Fiber 8.7 g Sugar 9.2 g Protein 9.7 g

Beet & Strawberry Smoothie

Preparation time: 10 minutes

Servings: 2

Ingredients:

- 2 cups frozen strawberries, pitted and chopped
- ⅔ cup roasted and frozen beet, chopped
- 1 teaspoon fresh ginger, peeled and grated
- 1 teaspoon fresh turmeric, peeled and grated
- ½ cup fresh orange juice
- 1 cup unsweetened almond milk

Directions:

1. Place all the Ingredients: in a high-speed blender and pulse until creamy.
2. Pour the smoothie into two glasses and serve immediately.

Nutrition: Calories 258 Total Fat 1.5 g Saturated Fat 0.1 g Cholesterol 0 mg Sodium 134 mg Total Carbs 26.7g Fiber 4.9 g Sugar 18.7 g Protein 2.9 g

---

Kiwi Smoothie

Preparation time: 10 minutes

Servings: 2

Ingredients:

- 4 kiwis
- 2 small bananas, peeled
- 1½ cups unsweetened almond milk
- 1-2 drops liquid stevia
- ¼ cup ice cubes

Directions:

1. Place all the Ingredients: in a high-speed blender and pulse until creamy.
2. Pour the smoothie into two glasses and serve immediately.

Nutrition: Calories 228 Total Fat 3.8 g Saturated Fat 0.4 g Cholesterol 0 mg Sodium 141 mg Total Carbs 50.7 g Fiber 8.4 g Sugar 28.1 g Protein 3.8 g

Pineapple & Carrot Smoothie

Preparation time: 10 minutes

Servings: 2

Ingredients:

- 1 cup frozen pineapple
- 1 large ripe banana, peeled and sliced
- ½ tablespoon fresh ginger, peeled and chopped
- ¼ teaspoon ground turmeric
- 1 cup unsweetened almond milk
- ½ cup fresh carrot juice
- 1 tablespoon fresh lemon juice

Directions:

1. Place all the Ingredients: in a high-speed blender and pulse until creamy.
2. Pour the smoothie into two glasses and serve immediately.

Nutrition: Calories 132 Total Fat 2.2 g Saturated Fat 0.3 g Cholesterol 0 mg Sodium 113 mg Total Carbs 629.3 g Fiber 4.1 g Sugar 16.9 g Protein 2 g

---

Oats & Orange Smoothie

Preparation time: 10 minutes

Servings: 4

Ingredients:

- ⅔ cup rolled oats
- 2 oranges, peeled, seeded, and sectioned
- 2 large bananas, peeled and sliced
- 2 cups unsweetened almond milk
- 1 cup ice cubes, crushed

Directions:

1. Place all the Ingredients: in a high-speed blender and pulse until creamy.
2. Pour the smoothie into four glasses and serve immediately.

Nutrition: Calories 175 ;Total Fat 3 g Saturated Fat 0.4 g Cholesterol 0 mg Sodium 93 mg Total Carbs 36.6 g Fiber 5.9 g Sugar 17.1 g Protein 3.9 g

Pumpkin Smoothie

Preparation time: 10 minutes

Servings: 2

Ingredients:

- 1 cup homemade pumpkin puree
- 1 medium banana, peeled and sliced
- 1 tablespoon maple syrup
- 1 teaspoon ground flaxseeds
- ½ teaspoon ground cinnamon
- ¼ teaspoon ground ginger
- 1½ cups unsweetened almond milk
- ¼ cup ice cubes

Directions:

1. Place all the Ingredients: in a high-speed blender and pulse until creamy.
2. Pour the smoothie into two glasses and serve immediately.

Nutrition: Calories 159 Total Fat 3.6 g Saturated Fat 0.5 g Cholesterol 0 mg Sodium 143 mg Total Carbs 32.6 g Fiber 6.5 g Sugar 17.3 g Protein 3 g

Red Veggie & Fruit Smoothie

Preparation time: 10 minutes

Servings: 2

Ingredients:

- ½ cup fresh raspberries
- ½ cup fresh strawberries
- ½ red bell pepper, seeded and chopped
- ½ cup red cabbage, chopped
- 1 small tomato
- 1 cup water
- ½ cup ice cubes

Directions:

1. Place all the Ingredients: in a high-speed blender and pulse until creamy.
2. Pour the smoothie into two glasses and serve immediately.

Nutrition: Calories 39 Cholesterol 0 mg Saturated Fat 0 g Sodium 10 mg Total Carbs 8.9 g Fiber 3.5 g Sugar 4.8 g Protein 1.3 g Total Fat 0.4 g

Kale Smoothie

Preparation time: 10 minutes

Servings: 2

Ingredients:

- 3 stalks fresh kale, trimmed and chopped
- 1-2 celery stalks, chopped
- ½ avocado, peeled, pitted, and chopped
- ½-inch piece ginger root, chopped
- ½-inch piece turmeric root, chopped
- 2 cups coconut milk

Directions:

1. Place all the Ingredients: in a high-speed blender and pulse until creamy.
2. Pour the smoothie into two glasses and serve immediately.

Nutrition: Calories 248 Total Fat 21.8 g Saturated Fat 12 g Cholesterol 0 mg Sodium 59 mg Total Carbs 11.3 g Fiber 4.2 g Sugar 0.5 g Protein 3.5 g

---

Green Tofu Smoothie

Preparation time: 10 minutes

Servings: 2

Ingredients:

- 1½ cups cucumber, peeled and chopped roughly
- 3 cups fresh baby spinach
- 2 cups frozen broccoli
- ½ cup silken tofu, drained and pressed
- 1 tablespoon fresh lime juice
- 4-5 drops liquid stevia
- 1 cup unsweetened almond milk
- ½ cup ice, crushed

Directions:

1. Place all the Ingredients: in a high-speed blender and pulse until creamy.
2. Pour the smoothie into two glasses and serve immediately.

Nutrition: Calories 118 Total Fat 15 g Saturated Fat 0.8 g Cholesterol 0 mg Sodium 165 mg Total Carbs 12.6 g Fiber 4.8 g Sugar 3.4 g Protein 10 g

Grape & Swiss Chard Smoothie

Preparation time: 10 minutes

Servings: 2

Ingredients:

- 2 cups seedless green grapes
- 2 cups fresh Swiss chard, trimmed and chopped
- 2 tablespoons maple syrup
- 1 teaspoon fresh lemon juice
- 1½ cups water
- 4 ice cubes

Directions:

1. Place all the Ingredients: in a high-speed blender and pulse until creamy.
2. Pour the smoothie into two glasses and serve immediately.

Nutrition: Calories 176 Total Fat 0.2 g Saturated Fat 0 g Cholesterol 0 mg Sodium 83 mg Total Carbs 44.9 g Fiber 1.7 g Sugar 37.9 g Protein 0.7 g

Matcha Smoothie

Preparation time: 10 minutes

Servings: 2

Ingredients:

- 2 tablespoons chia seeds
- 2 teaspoons matcha green tea powder
- ½ teaspoon fresh lemon juice
- ½ teaspoon xanthan gum
- 8-10 drops liquid stevia
- 4 tablespoons coconut cream
- 1½ cups unsweetened almond milk
- ¼ cup ice cubes

Directions:

1. Place all the **Ingredients:** in a high-speed blender and pulse until creamy.
2. Pour the smoothie into two glasses and serve immediately.

Nutrition: Calories 132 Total Fat 12.3 g Saturated Fat 6.8 g Cholesterol 0 mg Sodium 15 mg Total Carbs 7 g Fiber 4.8 g Sugar 1 g Protein 3 g

Banana Smoothie

Preparation time: 10 minutes

Servings: 2

Ingredients:

- 2 cups chilled unsweetened almond milk
- 1 large frozen banana, peeled and sliced
- 1 tablespoon almonds, chopped
- 1 teaspoon organic vanilla extract

Directions:

1. Place all the Ingredients: in a high-speed blender and pulse until creamy.
2. Pour the smoothie into two glasses and serve immediately.

Nutrition: Calories 124 Total Fat 5.2 g Saturated Fat 0.5 g Cholesterol 0 mg Sodium 181 mg Total Carbs 18.4 g Fiber 3.1 g Sugar 8.7 g Protein 2.4 g

---

Strawberry Smoothie

Ingredients:

- 2 cups chilled unsweetened almond milk
- 1½ cups frozen strawberries
- 1 banana, peeled and sliced
- ¼ teaspoon organic vanilla extract

Directions:

1. Add all the Ingredients: in a high-speed blender and pulse until smooth.
2. Pour the smoothie into two glasses and serve immediately.

Preparation time: 10 minutes

Servings: 2

Nutrition: Calories 131 Total Fat 3.7 g Saturated Fat 0.4 g Cholesterol 0 mg Sodium 181 mg Total Carbs 25.3 g Fiber 4.8 g Sugar 14 g Protein 1.6 g

Raspberry & Tofu Smoothie

Preparation time: 15 minutes

Servings: 2

Ingredients:

- 1½ cups fresh raspberries
- 6 ounces firm silken tofu, drained
- 1/8 teaspoon coconut extract
- 1 teaspoon powdered stevia
- 1½ cups unsweetened almond milk
- ¼ cup ice cubes, crushed

Directions:

1. Add all the Ingredients: in a high-speed blender and pulse until smooth.
2. Pour the smoothie into two glasses and serve immediately.

Nutrition: Calories 131 Total Fat 5.5 g Saturated Fat 0.6 g Cholesterol 0 mg Sodium 167 mg Total Carbs 14.6 g Fiber 6.8 g Sugar 5.2 g Protein 7.7 g

---

Mango Smoothie

Preparation time: 10 minutes

Servings: 2

Ingredients:

- 2 cups frozen mango, peeled, pitted and chopped
- ¼ cup almond butter
- Pinch of ground turmeric
- 2 tablespoons fresh lemon juice
- 1¼ cups unsweetened almond milk
- ¼ cup ice cubes

Directions:

1. Add all the Ingredients: in a high-speed blender and pulse until smooth.
2. Pour the smoothie into two glasses and serve immediately.

Nutrition: Calories 140 Total Fat 4.1 g Saturated Fat 0.6 g Cholesterol 0 mg Sodium 118 mg Total Carbs 26.8 g Fiber 3.6 g Sugar 23 g Protein 2.5 g

Pineapple Smoothie

Preparation time: 10 minutes

Servings: 2

Ingredients:

- 2 cups pineapple, chopped
- ½ teaspoon fresh ginger, peeled and chopped
- ½ teaspoon ground turmeric
- 1 teaspoon natural immune support supplement *
- 1 teaspoon chia seeds
- 1½ cups cold green tea
- ½ cup ice, crushed

Directions:

1. Add all the Ingredients: in a high-speed blender and pulse until smooth.
2. Pour the smoothie into two glasses and serve immediately.

Nutrition: Calories 152 Total Fat 1 g Saturated Fat 0 g Cholesterol 0 mg Sodium 9 mg Total Carbs 30 g Fiber 3.5 g Sugar 29.8 g Protein 1.5 g

*note: this supplement is packed with about 20-25 proteins, vitamins, herbs and superfoods that boost the immune system of the body.

Kale & Pineapple Smoothie

Preparation time: 15 minutes

Servings: 2

Ingredients:

- 1½ cups fresh kale, trimmed and chopped
- 1 frozen banana, peeled and chopped
- ½ cup fresh pineapple chunks
- 1 cup unsweetened coconut milk
- ½ cup fresh orange juice
- ½ cup ice

Directions:

1. Add all the Ingredients: in a high-speed blender and pulse until smooth.
2. Pour the smoothie into two glasses and serve immediately.

Nutrition: Calories 148 Total Fat 2.4 g Saturated Fat 2.1 g Cholesterol 0 mg Sodium 23 mg Total Carbs 31.6 g Fiber 3.5 g Sugar 16.5 g Protein 2.8 g

Green Veggies Smoothie

Preparation time: 15 minutes

Servings: 2

Ingredients:

- 1 medium avocado, peeled, pitted, and chopped
- 1 large cucumber, peeled and chopped
- 2 fresh tomatoes, chopped
- 1 small green bell pepper, seeded and chopped
- 1 cup fresh spinach, torn
- 2 tablespoons fresh lime juice
- 2 tablespoons homemade vegetable broth
- 1 cup alkaline water

Directions:

1. Add all the Ingredients: in a high-speed blender and pulse until smooth.
2. Pour the smoothie into glasses and serve immediately.

Nutrition: Calories 275 Total Fat 20.3 g Saturated Fat 4.2 g Cholesterol 0 mg Sodium 76 mg Total Carbs 24.1 g Fiber 10.1 g Sugar 9.3 g Protein 5.3 g

---

Avocado & Spinach Smoothie

Preparation time: 10 minutes

Servings: 2

Ingredients:

- 2 cups fresh baby spinach
- ½ avocado, peeled, pitted, and chopped
- 4-6 drops liquid stevia
- ½ teaspoon ground cinnamon
- 1 tablespoon hemp seeds
- 2 cups chilled alkaline water

Directions:

1. Add all the Ingredients: in a high-speed blender and pulse until smooth.
2. Pour the smoothie into two glasses and serve immediately.

Nutrition: Calories 132 Total Fat 11.7 g Saturated Fat 2.2 g Cholesterol 0 mg Sodium 27 mg Total Carbs 6.1 g Fiber 4.5 g Sugar 0.4 g Protein 3.1 g

Cucumber Smoothie

Preparation time: 15 minutes

Servings: 2

Ingredients:

- 1 small cucumber, peeled and chopped
- 2 cups mixed fresh greens (spinach, kale, beet greens), trimmed and chopped
- ½ cup lettuce, torn
- ¼ cup fresh parsley leaves
- ¼ cup fresh mint leaves
- 2-3 drops liquid stevia
- 1 teaspoon fresh lemon juice
- 1½ cups filtered water
- ¼ cup ice cubes

Directions:

1. Add all the Ingredients: in a high-speed blender and pulse until smooth.
2. Pour the smoothie into two glasses and serve immediately.

Nutrition: Calories 50 Total Fat 0.5 g Saturated Fat 0.2 g Cholesterol 0 mg Sodium 34 mg Total Carbs 11.3 g Fiber 3.6 g Sugar 3.2 g Protein 2.5 g

---

Apple Ginger Smoothie

Preparation time: 10 minutes

Cooking time: 0 minutes

Servings: 01

Ingredients:

- 1 Apple, peeled and diced
- ¾ cup (6 oz) coconut yogurt
- ½ teaspoon ginger, freshly grated

Directions:

1. Add all the Ingredients: to a blender.
2. Blend well until smooth.
3. Refrigerate for 2 to 3 hours.
4. Serve.

Nutrition: Calories 144 Total Fat 0.4 g Saturated Fat 5 g Cholesterol 51 mg Sodium 86 mg Total Carbs 8 g Fiber 2.3 g Sugar 2.2 g Protein 5.6 g

Green Tea Blueberry Smoothie

Preparation time: 10 minutes

Cooking time: 5 minutes

Servings: 01

Ingredients:

- 3 tablespoons alkaline water
- 1 green tea bag
- 1½ cup fresh blueberries
- 1 pear, peeled, cored and diced
- ¾ cup almond milk

Directions:

1. Boil 3 tablespoons water in a small pot and transfer it to a cup.
2. Dip the tea bag in the cup and let it sit for 4 to 5 mins.
3. Discard tea bag and
4. Transfer the green tea to a blender
5. Add all the remaining the Ingredients: to the blender.
6. Blend well until smooth.
7. Serve with fresh blueberries.

Nutrition: Calories 144 Total Fat 0.4 g Saturated Fat 5 g Cholesterol 51 mg Sodium 86 mg Total Carbs 8 g Fiber 2.3 g Sugar 2.2 g Protein 5.6 g

---

Apple Almond Smoothie

Preparation time: 10 minutes

Cooking time: 0 minutes

Servings: 01

Ingredients:

- 1 cup apple cider
- 1/2 cup coconut yogurt
- 4 tablespoons almonds, crushed
- 1/4 teaspoon cinnamon
- 1/4 teaspoon nutmeg
- 1 cup ice cubes

Directions:

1. Add all the Ingredients: to a blender.
2. Blend well until smooth.
3. Serve.

Nutrition: Calories 144 Total Fat 0.4 g Saturated Fat 5 g Cholesterol 51 mg Sodium 86 mg Total Carbs 8 g Fiber 2.3 g Sugar 2.2 g Protein 5.6 g

Cranberry Smoothie

Preparation time: 10 minutes

Cooking time: 0 minutes

Servings: 01

Ingredients:

- 1 cup cranberries
- ¾ cup almond milk
- ¼ cup raspberries
- 2 teaspoon fresh ginger, finely grated
- 2 teaspoons fresh lemon juice

Directions:

1. Add all the Ingredients: to a blender.
2. Blend well until smooth.
3. Serve with fresh berries on top.

Nutrition: Calories 144 Total Fat 0.4 g Saturated Fat 5 g Cholesterol 51 mg Sodium 86 mg Total Carbs 8 g Fiber 2.3 g Sugar 2.2 g Protein 5.6 g

---

Cinnamon Berry Smoothie

Preparation time: 10 minutes

Cooking time: 0 minutes

Servings: 01

Ingredients:

- 1 cup frozen strawberries
- 1 cup apple, peeled and diced
- 2 teaspoon fresh ginger
- 3 tablespoons hemp seeds
- 1 cup water
- ½ lime juiced
- ¼ teaspoon cinnamon powder
- ⅛ teaspoon vanilla extract

Directions:

1. Add all the Ingredients: to a blender.
2. Blend well until smooth.
3. Serve with fresh fruits

Nutrition: Calories 144 Total Fat 0.4 g Saturated Fat 5 g Cholesterol 51 mg Sodium 86 mg Total Carbs 8 g Fiber 2.3 g Sugar 2.2 g Protein 5.6 g

Detox Berries smoothie

Preparation time: 10 minutes

Cooking time: 0 minutes

Servings: 01

Ingredients:

- 3 peaches, cored and peeled
- 5 blueberries
- 5 raspberries
- 1 cup alkaline water

Directions:

1. Add all the Ingredients: to a blender.
2. Blend well until smooth.
3. Serve with fresh kiwi wedges.

Nutrition: Calories 144 Total Fat 0.4 g Saturated Fat 5 g Cholesterol 51 mg Sodium 86 mg Total Carbs 8 g Fiber 2.3 g Sugar 2.2 g Protein 5.6 g

Pink Smoothie

Preparation time: 10 minutes

Cooking time: 0 minutes

Servings: 01

Ingredients:

- 1 peach, cored and peeled
- 6 ripe strawberries
- 1 cup almond milk

Directions:

1. Add all the Ingredients: to a blender.
2. Blend well until smooth.
3. Serve with your favorite berries

Nutrition: Calories 144 Total Fat 0.4 g Saturated Fat 5 g Cholesterol 51 mg Sodium 86 mg Total Carbs 8 g Fiber 2.3 g Sugar 2.2 g Protein 5.6 g

Green Apple Smoothie

Preparation time: 10 minutes

Cooking time: 0 minutes

Servings: 01

Ingredients:

- 1 peach , peeled and cored
- 1 green apple, peeled and cored
- 1 cup alkaline water

Directions:

1. Add all the Ingredients: to a blender.
2. Blend well until smooth.
3. Serve with apple slices.

Nutrition:

Calories 144 Total Fat 0.4 g Saturated Fat 5 g Cholesterol 51 mg Sodium 86 mg Total Carbs 8 g Fiber 2.3 g Sugar 2.2 g Protein 5.6 g

---

Avocado Smoothie

Preparation time: 10 minutes

Cooking time: 0 minutes

Servings: 01

Ingredients:

- 1 carrot, grated
- 1 avocado, cored and peeled
- ½ pear, cored
- ½ cup blackberries
- 1 ½ cups unsweetened almond milk

Directions:

1. Add all the Ingredients: to a blender.
2. Blend well until smooth.
3. Serve with blackberries on top.

Nutrition:

Calories 144 Total Fat 0.4 g Saturated Fat 5 g Cholesterol 51 mg Sodium 86 mg Total Carbs 8 g Fiber 2.3 g Sugar 2.2 g Protein 5.6 g

Green Smoothie

Preparation time: 10 minutes

Cooking time: 0 minutes

Servings: 01

Ingredients:

- 1 cup alkaline water
- 3/4 cup raw coconut water
- 1/2 teaspoon probiotic powder
- 2 cups firmly packed baby spinach
- 1 cup raw young Thai coconut meat
- 1 avocado, peeled and pitted
- 1/2 cucumber, chopped-chopped
- 1 teaspoon lime zest, finely grated
- 2 limes, hav
- led
- Stevia, to taste
- Pinch of Celtic sea salt
- 2 cups ice cubes

Directions:

1. Add all the Ingredients: to a blender.
2. Blend well until smooth.
3. Serve with an avocado slice on top.

Nutrition: Calories 144 Total Fat 0.4 g Saturated Fat 5 g Cholesterol 51 mg Sodium 86 mg Total Carbs 8 g Fiber 2.3 g Sugar 2.2 g Protein 5.6 g

---

Oats & Orange Smoothie

Preparation time: 10 minutes.

Servings: 4

Ingredients:

- 2/3 cups rolled oats
- 2 oranges, peeled, seeded, and sectioned
- 2 large bananas, peeled and sliced
- 2 cups unsweetened almond milk
- 1 cup ice cubes, crushed

Directions:

1. Place all the Ingredients: in a high-speed blender and pulse until creamy.
2. Pour the smoothie into four glasses and serve immediately.

Nutrition: Total Fat 3 g; Saturated Fat 0.4 g; Sodium 93 mg; Total Carbs 36.6 g; Fiber 5.9 g; Sugar 11.7 g; Protein 5.9 g; Calories 175; Cholesterol 0 mg

Spiced Banana Smoothie

Preparation time: 5 minutes. Total time: 5 minutes

Servings: 2

Ingredients:

- 2 medium frozen bananas, peeled and sliced
- 1 tsp organic vanilla extract
- ¼ tsp ground cinnamon
- Pinch of ground nutmeg
- Pinch of ground cloves
- 1½ cups unsweetened almond milk

Directions:

1. Place all the Ingredients: in a high-speed blender and pulse until creamy.
2. Pour the smoothie into two glasses and serve immediately.

Nutrition: Calories 143; Total Fat 2.1 g; Saturated Fat 0.4 g; Sodium 137 mg; Fiber 4 g; Sugar 14.8 g; Protein 2.1 g; Cholesterol 0 mg; Total Carbs 29.1 g

---

Blueberry Smoothie

Preparation time: 5 minutes. Total time: 5 minutes

Servings: 2

Ingredients:

- 2 cups frozen blueberries
- 1½ cups unsweetened almond milk
- 1 small banana, peeled and sliced
- ¼ cup ice cubes

Directions:

1. Place all the Ingredients: in a high-speed blender and pulse until creamy.
2. Serve immediately after pouring the smoothie into two glasses.

Nutrition: Calories 158; Saturated Fat 0.3 g; Sodium 137 mg; Total Carbs 34 g; Fiber 5.6 g; Sugar 20 g; Protein 2.2 g; Total Fat 3.3 g; Cholesterol 0 mg

Raspberry & Tofu Smoothie

Preparation time: 10 minutes.

Servings: 2

Ingredients:

- 8 oz firm silken tofu, pressed and drained
- 1 cup frozen raspberries
- ¼ tsp coconut extract
- 4-6 drops liquid stevia
- 1 cup coconut cream
- ½ cup ice cubes, crushed

Directions:

1. Place all the Ingredients: in a high-speed blender and pulse until creamy.
2. Pour the smoothie into two glasses and serve immediately.

Nutrition: Calories 328; Saturated Fat 9.7 g; Sodium 32 mg; Total Carbs 39.4 g; Fiber 6.5 g; Sugar 28 g; Protein 11.4g; Total Fat 15.4 g; Cholesterol 0 mg

Papaya Smoothie

Preparation time: 10 minutes.

Servings: 2

Ingredients:

- 1 large banana, peeled and sliced
- ½ medium papaya, peeled and chopped roughly
- 1½ cups unsweetened almond milk
- 2 tbsp agave syrup
- 1 tbsp fresh lime juice
- ¼ tsp ground turmeric
- ½ cup ice cubes, crushed

Directions:

1. Place all the Ingredients: in a high-speed blender and pulse until creamy.
2. Pour the smoothie into two glasses and serve immediately.

Nutrition: Calories 190; Total Fat 3.1 g; Saturated Fat 0.4 g; Sodium 157 mg; Total Carbs 42.6 g; Sugar 14.5 g; Protein 1.9 g; Cholesterol 0 mg; Fiber 3.9 g

Peach Smoothie

Preparation time: 10 minutes.

Servings: 2

Ingredients:

- 1 large peach, peeled, pitted, and chopped
- 1 medium frozen banana, peeled and sliced
- 2 oz aloe vera
- ½ tsp fresh ginger, peeled and chopped
- 2 tbsp flax seeds
- ½ tsp organic vanilla extract
- 1¾ cups unsweetened almond milk

Directions:

1. Add all the Ingredients: in a high-speed blender and pulse until smooth.
2. Pour the smoothie into two glasses and serve immediately.

Nutrition: Calories 162; Saturated Fat 0.6 g; Sodium 160 mg; Total Carbs 25.7g; Fiber 5.5 g; Sugar 14.5 g; Protein 3.6 g; Cholesterol 0 mg; Total Fat 5.7 g

---

Strawberry & Beet Smoothie

Preparation time: 10 minutes.

Servings: 2

Ingredients:

- 2 cups frozen strawberries, pitted and chopped
- 2/3 cup frozen beets, chopped
- 1 tsp fresh ginger, peeled and grated
- 1 tsp fresh turmeric, peeled and grated
- ½ cup fresh orange juice
- 1 cup unsweetened almond milk

Directions:

1. Add all the Ingredients: in a high-speed blender and pulse until smooth.
2. Pour the smoothie into two glasses and serve immediately.

Nutrition: Calories 130; Saturated Fat 0.2 g; Sodium 135 mg; Total Carbs 27.5 g; Fiber 5.1 g; Sugar 18.7 g; Protein 2 g; Cholesterol 0 mg; Total Fat 2.1 g

Grape & Swiss Chard Smoothie

Preparation time: 10 minutes.

Servings: 2

Ingredients:

- 2 cups seedless green grapes
- 2 cups fresh Swiss chard, trimmed and chopped
- 2 tbsp agave nectar
- 1 tsp fresh lemon juice
- 1½ cups alkaline water
- ¼ cup ice cubes, crushed

Directions:

1. Add all the Ingredients: in a high-speed blender and pulse until smooth.
2. Pour the smoothie into two glasses and serve immediately.

Nutrition: Calories 128; Saturated Fat 0 g; Sodium 78 mg; Total Carbs 33.4 g; Fiber 2.6 g; Sugar 30.5 g; Protein 1.7g; Cholesterol 0 mg; Total Fat 1.1 g

---

Kale Smoothie

Preparation time: 10 minutes.

Servings: 2

Ingredients:

- 1 cup fresh kale, tough ribs removed and chopped
- 1-2 celery stalks, chopped
- ½ avocado, peeled, pitted, and chopped
- ½-1 ginger root, chopped
- ½ turmeric root, chopped
- 1½ cups unsweetened coconut milk
- ¼ cup ice cubes, crushed

Directions:

1. Add all the Ingredients: in a high-speed blender and pulse until smooth.
2. Pour the smoothie into two glasses and serve immediately.

Nutrition: Calories 158; Saturated Fat 5.1 g; Sodium 26 mg; Total Carbs 10.3 g; Fiber 4.9 g; Sugar 0.4 g; Protein 2.1 g; Cholesterol 0 mg; Total Fat 12.9 g

Green Veggie Smoothie

Preparation time: 10 minutes.

Servings: 2

Ingredients:

- ½ small cucumber, peeled and chopped roughly
- 1 cup fresh dandelion greens, chopped
- 1 celery stalk, chopped
- ¼ tsp fresh ginger, chopped
- 8-10 drops liquid stevia
- ½ tbsp fresh lime juice
- 1½ cups alkaline water
- ¼ cup ice cubes, crushed

Directions:

1. Add all the Ingredients: in a high-speed blender and pulse until smooth.
2. Pour the smoothie into two glasses and serve immediately.

Nutrition: Calories 26; Saturated Fat 0.1 g; Sodium 30 mg; Total Carbs 5.7 g; Fiber 1.5 g; Sugar 1.6 g; Protein 1.3 g; Cholesterol 0 mg; Total Fat 0.3 g

---

Pepper Mint Tea Surprise

Prep time: 4 minutes, Cook time: 15 minutes

Serves: 2

Ingredients:

- 1 tablespoon peppermint leaves
- 1 tablespoon regular mint
- 1 tablespoon basil leaves
- A few dates, pitted
- 2 cups alkaline water

Directions:

1. Boil the water.
2. Place the tea Ingredients: and the dates in a tea pot or tea cup.
3. Pour over some boiling water and cover.
4. Leave covered for 15 minutes.
5. Strain all the Ingredients: and serve in a nice tea cup.
6. Feel free to throw in the dates back (yummy!). You can also re-use them to make a smoothie, using some of the recipes in this book that call for dates.

Chamomile Tea with Parsley

Prep time: 3 minutes, Cook time: 15 minutes

Serves: 2

Ingredients:

- 2 tablespoons chamomile flowers
- 2 tablespoons parsley
- 2 cups alkaline water
- A few mint leaves to garnish

Directions:

1. Boil the water.
2. Place the tea Ingredients: in a tea pot or tea cup.
3. Pour over the boiling water and cover.
4. Leave covered for 15 minutes.
5. Strain all the Ingredients: and serve in a nice tea cup.
6. Garnish with some mint leaves.
7. Enjoy!

Lavender Mint Tea

Prep time: 5 minutes, Cook time: 5 minutes

Serves: 2-4

Ingredients:

- 2 tablespoons lavender flowers
- 2 tablespoons mint leaves
- 4 cups alkaline water

Directions:

1. Clean the lavender flowers thoroughly under running water.
2. Chop it roughly and place it in a large saucepan.
3. Clean and roughly chop the mint leaves and add to the saucepan.
4. Add the water to the pan and allow it to come to a boil.
5. Once it starts to boil, lower the heat and simmer for 5 minutes.
6. Strain and pour into a mug.
7. Serve and enjoy!

Almond Milk and Rosemary Tea

Prep time: 2 minutes, Cook time: 5 minutes

Serves: 2

Ingredients:

- 2 cups almond milk
- 4 tablespoons rosemary herb
- A few banana slices
- A few apple slices
- 1 tablespoon coconut oil

Directions:

1. Heat the almond milk in a saucepan.
2. Place the rest of the Ingredients: in a tea pot or a tea cup.
3. Pour over the boiling milk.
4. Cover for 15 minutes.
5. Strain and pour into a tea cup.
6. Enjoy!

Cucumber Infused Lemon Iced Tea

Prep time: 8 minutes, Cook time: 10 minutes

Serves: 2-3

Ingredients:

- 2 cups cucumber
- 3 cups alkaline water
- 1 cup lemon juice
- Stevia to sweeten (optional)
- Ice cubes
- Mint leaves

Directions:

1. Boil one cup of water.
2. Clean the cucumber thoroughly and remove the pith from both ends.
3. Cut it into thin circles or little pieces.
4. Place it in a bowl and add stevia (optional).
5. Pour the hot water on top and allow it to rest for 10 minutes.
6. Meanwhile, mix the two cups of water and the lemon juice and place it in the fridge.
7. Crush the ice in a coffee grinder or blender.
8. Strain the cucumber water and add the ice cubes.
9. Add in the cold lemon juice. Sprinkle some roughly chopped mint leaves on top and serve.

Nice and Fresh Mint Smoothie

This smoothie is great for digestion and is full of antioxidant properties. In addition, it helps you keep hydrated and nicely refreshed. Personally, I find the mint really effective in alleviating headaches and staying energized naturally without having to resort to caffeine.

Servings: 1

Ingredients:

- Half cup of frozen or fresh blueberries
- 1 cup of fresh chopped spinach
- 1 cup of unsweetened almond milk or coconut milk
- 2 tablespoons of fresh chopped mint
- 1 teaspoon of stevia or a few banana slices
- Optional (to garnish):
- -a few mint leaves
- -a slice of lime

Instructions:

1. Combine the spinach and almond milk in a high-speed blender.
2. Blend well until smooth and add the rest of the Ingredients:.
3. Blend again to make sure there are no lumps.
4. Pour your smoothie into a glass and enjoy right away.

Simple Raspberry Smoothie

Ever since I was a kid, I loved raspberries. It's one of my favourite fruits and whenever I can get it (I stick to seasonal options only) I turn them into smoothies. This one is miraculous and if you can combine it with some green powders you will create a nourishing green smoothie that is very tempting (great for green smoothie beginners). It's all about balance.

Serves: 1-2

Ingredients:

- 1 cup raspberries (you could also use blueberries)
- 1 cup almond milk or coconut milk
- Juice of 2 grapefruits
- Pinch of Himalayan salt
- Optional: 1 teaspoon of alfalfa or barley grass powder

Instructions:

1. Simply blend and serve.
2. Enjoy!

Refreshing Green Smoothie

Smoothies are always a great way to start your day and they are super quick to make. One smoothie a day will keep the doctor a way and it's better to schedule it first thing in the morning, before you get too busy.

Servings: 1 to 2

Ingredients:

- A few pineapple slices
- ½ cup baby spinach
- 1 cup coconut milk
- 6 to 8 ice cubes
- 1 teaspoon alfalfa powder or barley grass
- Juice of 2 limes

Instructions:

1. Combine the smoothie Ingredients: in a blender.
2. Blend until smooth and then add in the lime juice.
3. Pour your smoothie into a glass, drink and enjoy!

Sweet Cherry and Chia Smoothie

Servings: 1 to 2

Ingredients:

- ½ cup of frozen or fresh cherries
- ½ cup baby spinach
- 1 cup of almond milk
- 2 tablespoons of raw chia seeds
- Pinch ground ginger

Instructions:

1. Combine the smoothie Ingredients: in a blender.
2. First blend the spinach and cherries.
3. Add the milk, chia seeds and ginger.
4. Pour your finished smoothie into glasses and drink.

Spinach Green Tea Energy Smoothie

While caffeine in all its forms is not really alkaline, there is nothing wrong with an occasional cup of tea, especially green tea that is full of antioxidants and fat-burning properties. Great in a smoothie!

Servings: 2-3

Ingredients:

- 1 cup chopped baby spinach
- 1 small ripe avocado
- 1 cup brewed green tea, chilled
- Juice of 2 grapefruits
- Stevia to sweeten (optional)

Instructions:

1. Combine the smoothie Ingredients: in a blender and process a few times until smooth.
2. Pour your finished smoothie into glasses and drink.

Fruity Spicy Tropical Smoothie

While most fruit (especially "sugary" fruit) is not super alkaline, fruit is totally okay as a part of a balanced diet. It's also much healthier than processed carbs or sugary treats. There is no doubt about it. The spices used in this smoothie have anti-inflammatory and alkalizing properties and the green tea will give you a boost of energy.

Servings: 2-3

Ingredients:

- 1 cup blueberries
- 1 cup fresh papaya, chopped
- 1 medium banana
- A few ice cubes
- 2 cups brewed green tea, chilled
- 1 teaspoon ground turmeric
- 1 teaspoon ground ginger
- 1 teaspoon ground ginger
- Pinch cayenne pepper
- Optional: stevia

Instructions:

1. Combine the smoothie Ingredients: in a blender.
2. Blend well until smooth and add the spices.
3. Pour your finished smoothie into glasses and drink.
4. Enjoy!

Leafy Green Smoothie

Here is another smoothie that combines detoxifying and energizing properties. It is great to start your day feeling amazing!

Servings: 1 to 2

Ingredients:

- 1 cup of chopped kale
- 1 medium green apple, cored and chopped
- 1 stalk of celery, chopped
- ¼ cup of fresh parsley, minced
- 1 cup of fresh pomegranate or grapefruit juice
- A few ice cubes
- 1 tablespoon hemp seeds
- Stevia to sweeten (optional)

Instructions:

1. Combine the smoothie Ingredients: in a blender.
2. Blend well until smooth.
3. Pour your finished smoothie into a glass and drink.
4. Enjoy!

Super Alkalizing Avocado Coconut Smoothie

Servings: 1 to 2

Ingredients:

- 2 cups fresh chopped baby spinach
- 1 small chopped avocado
- ¼ cup of fresh chopped cilantro
- 1 cup chilled coconut water
- 1 tablespoon grated ginger, fresh
- ½ teaspoon ground turmeric
- Pinch cayenne

Instructions:

1. Combine the smoothie Ingredients: in your high-speed blender.
2. Pulse the Ingredients: a few times to chop them up.
3. Blend the mixture on the highest speed setting for 30 to 60 seconds.
4. Pour your finished smoothie into glasses and drink.
5. Enjoy!

Hydrating Watermelon Smoothie

This smoothie is great on a warm, summer morning, or anytime during the day. Watermelon combined with coconut water offer hydration, rejuvenation and energy.

Servings: 2-3

Ingredients:

- 1 cup frozen blueberries
- 1 cup fresh chopped watermelon
- 1 inch fresh sliced ginger
- 1 cup coconut water
- 1 tablespoon raw chia seeds
- A few ice cubes

Instructions:

1. Combine the smoothie Ingredients: in a blender.
2. Blend well until smooth.
3. Pour your finished smoothie into glasses and drink. Enjoy!

Ginger Protein Energy Smoothie

Servings: 1 to 2

Ingredients:

- 1 cup of chopped kale
- 1 cup pomegranates
- 1 medium carrot, diced
- 1 inch fresh grated ginger
- 1 cup coconut water
- 1 scoop hemp protein powder

Instructions:

1. Combine the smoothie Ingredients: in a blender.
2. Blend well until smooth.
3. Pour your finished smoothie into glasses and drink.

Peach Sweetness Smoothie

Servings: 1 to 2

Ingredients:

- 2 peaches, peeled and pitted
- 1 cup of almond milk
- 6 to 8 ice cubes
- 2 tablespoons raw hemp seeds or powder
- 1 teaspoon ground ginger
- Juice of 2 lemons

Instructions:

1. Combine the smoothie Ingredients: in a blender.
2. Blend until smooth, add ginger, ice cubes and hemp seeds.
3. Pour your finished smoothies into glasses and drink.
4. Enjoy!

Cucumber Melon Smoothie

I love this recipe in the summer! Honeydew melon gives it a nice taste which is great for those who are not used to drinking green smoothies.

Servings: 2

Ingredients:

- 1 cup of chopped honeydew melon
- 1 cup cucumber, diced
- 1 cup coconut water
- 1 tablespoon of fresh mint
- 1 tablespoon cilantro
- Pinch of Himalayan salt
- Juice of 1 lime
- Chia seeds (optional)

Instructions:

1. Blend the smoothie Ingredients: in a blender or food processor.
2. Add Himalayan salt to taste, mix well and if you wish, stir in some chia seeds for more nutrition.
3. Enjoy!

Fennel Magic Alka-Juice

Serves: 1-2

Ingredients:

- 2 cups fennel, chopped
- 2 tablespoons fennel seeds + 1 divided
- 2 cups spinach
- 2 cups carrot slices
- 1 pear, peeled and sliced
- ½ cup lemon juice
- Ice cubes

Instructions:

1. Wash all Ingredients: well. Clean and chop.
2. Add all Ingredients: (fennel, spinach, carrots, pear) through juicer.
3. Mix in some lemon juice. Place in a tall glass

4. Serve with a sprinkling of fennel seeds on top and it is best served chilled.
5. Ice cubes, and ginger ice cubes work great with this juice.
6. Enjoy!

Sweet Grapefruit Easy Mix

Pressed for time and want to alkalize? This recipe is super easy and full of alkalinity!

Serves: 1-2

Ingredients:

- 2 grapefruits
- 1 cup coconut water
- 1 cup almond milk
- ½ lemon
- 1 teaspoon powdered ginger
- ¼ cup warm water (not boiling)

Instructions:

1. Combine the powdered ginger and warm water until dissolved.
2. Add the lemon and grapefruit juice.
3. Add the coconut water and almond milk.
4. Add ice cubes or ginger ice cubes.
5. Enjoy!

Kukicha Smoothie

Ever heard of kukicha? If not, make sure you put it on your alkaline shopping list. If yes, I hope the following recipe will help you come up with more ideas on your alkaline journey!

Serves: 2

Ingredients:

- 1 cup kukicha tea
- 1 cup coconut milk
- ½ cup spinach
- 1 banana
- 1 inch ginger
- A green apple
- ¼ cup almonds (soaked in water for 8 hours or more)
- Optional: juice of 1 lemon

Instructions:

1. Blend all the Ingredients: until smooth.
2. For more alkalinity, add some lemon juice.
3. Stir well, serve, and enjoy!

Nice'n Fresh Smoothie

Soy sprouts and alfalfa sprouts are great, not only in your salads and soups, but also in your smoothies. When combined with other healthy and alkalizing **Ingredients:**, they create amazing alkaline balance and taste.

Serves: 2

Ingredients:

- 2 cups almond milk (unsweetened)
- ½ cup soy sprouts
- ½ cup alfalfa sprouts
- 1 inch ginger
- ½ an avocado
- 1 green apple
- 1 tablespoon avocado oil or coconut oil
- stevia to sweeten (optional)

Instructions:

1. Combine all the Ingredients:, except for oils, in a blender.
2. Blend until smooth.
3. Add some coconut oil or avocado oil. If you wish, sweeten with some stevia.
4. Enjoy!

Wake Up Maca Juice

Green, alkaline juices are natural energy boosters; however, by adding some maca powder, we can really take it to the next level!

Servings: 2-3

Ingredients:

- 1/2 cup water cress
- 3 big tomatoes
- A few fennel slices
- ½ inch ginger
- ½ cup parsley
- Juice of 1 lemon
- ½ teaspoon of maca powder
- 1 tablespoon olive oil or avocado oil

Procedure:

1. Wash and chop all the veggies.
2. Place through a juicer.
3. Place the juice in a tall glass and add some maca powder and lemon juice.
4. Add some olive or avocado oil for better absorption.

Additional Information:

Maca

This natural supplement is rich in Vitamin C, B, and E, as well as zinc, iron, calcium, magnesium, phosphorus, and amino acids. It has hormone balancing properties and acts as an aphrodisiac, both for men and women. As far as female health is concerned, maca can help alleviate menstrual cramps, as well as menopause issues (mood swings, depression, and anxiety).

Contraindications: avoid maca if pregnant or lactating. If on medication or suffering from any serious health problems, remember to contact your doctor first.

When trying maca for the first time, use no more than ½ teaspoon a day and go from there. The recommended maximum intake is actually about 1 teaspoon a day. However, remember that maca acts as a stimulant. Listen to your body; sometimes less is better.

Boost Your Metabolism Juice

This recipe offers a unique taste, pH balancing properties, metabolism boosting properties, and is also great for your skin.

Servings: 1-2

Ingredients:

- 1 cup fresh spinach
- 1 large grapefruit, juiced
- 1 carrot, small
- 2 celery stalks
- 1 beet
- ½ teaspoon cinnamon
- 1/2 inch of fresh stem ginger
- ¼ cup fresh mint leaves
- 1 tablespoon chia seeds

Procedure:

1. Wash the spinach, mint, grapefruit, carrot, celery stalks, and beet.
2. Chop the spinach, carrot (no need to peel if organic), celery, and beet.
3. Place through a juicer. While the juicer is working, you may juice the grapefruit (I use a simple lemon squeezer).
4. Mix the fresh veggie juice with grapefruit juice.
5. Add some chia seeds and stir well.
6. Drink immediately.
7. Enjoy!

Purple Energy Detox Juice

Beet root is extremely good for cleansing the liver. While I do agree it might not be the best juice for beginners, I can also tell you it's worth getting used to it. The juice is jam-packed with minerals and great for shedding unwanted pounds, not to mention higher energy levels! Lemon and lime juice add more flavor to this juice and make it a great, refreshing drink for any time of the day.

Servings: 1-2

Ingredients:

- 2 celery stalks
- 2 medium cucumbers
- ¼ cup parsley
- ¼ cup mint
- beet root
- 1 lemon, juiced
- 1 lime, juiced
- 1 tsp olive oil
- Pinch of Himalayan salt

Procedure:

1. Wash and chop all the Ingredients:.
2. Place celery, cucumbers, parsley, mint and beet root through a juicer.
3. When ready, place the juice in a juice glass or another utensil of your choice and stir in some lemon and lime juice, as well as Himalayan salt and a bit of olive oil (or any other quality cold-pressed oil) of your choice. Oils help your body with nutrient absorption. Enjoy!

Chapter 9. Condiments, Sauces & Dressings

Homemade Ketchup

Prep time: 5 minutes

Cooking time: 10 minutes

Servings: 2

Ingredients:

- 6-oz can unsweetened tomato paste
- ½ cup brown rice syrup
- ½ cup apple cider vinegar
- 1 packet stevia
- ¼ tsp onion powder
- ⅛ tsp garlic powder

Instructions:

1. In a saucepan over medium heat, combine all **Ingredients:**. Whisk until smooth.
2. Bring the mixture to a boil. Then simmer for 25 minutes, stirring frequently.
3. Chill and serve cold.
4. Nutrients per serving: Carbohydrates – 38.5 g Fiber – 2.7 g Fat – 3.5 g Protein – 11.7 g Calories – 172

Salsa Fresca

Prep time: 20 minutes

Cooking time: 0 minutes

Servings: 6

Ingredients:

- 4 fully ripened tomatoes, diced
- ½ sweet onion , diced
- tbsp cumin seeds, toasted
- ¼ cup fresh cilantro, chopped
- ¼ cup apple cider vinegar
- ½ tsp sea salt

Instructions:

1. In a large airtight container, mix together all Ingredients:.
2. Cover and chill for 15 minutes, so the flavors blend before serving.
3. Nutrients per serving: Carbohydrates – 4.6 g Fiber – 1.2 g Fat – 0.4 g Protein – 1.5 g Calories – 25

Hawaiian Salsa

Prep time: 20 minutes

Cooking time: 0 minutes

Servings: 6

Ingredients:

- 4 fully ripened tomatoes, diced
- ½ sweet onion, diced
- ½ cup fresh mango, diced
- ½ cup pineapple, diced
- ¼ cup apple cider vinegar
- ½ tsp sea salt

Instructions:

1. In a large airtight container, mix together all Ingredients:.
2. Cover and chill for 15 minutes so the flavors blend before serving.
3. Nutrients per serving: Carbohydrates – 5.3 g Fiber – 1.4 g Fat – 0.2 g Protein – 0.9 g Calories – 48

Great Gravy

Prep time: 5 minutes

Cooking time: 10 minutes

Servings: 6

Ingredients:

- Tbsp coconut oil, melted
- Tbsp coconut flour
- ½ cup vegetable broth
- Tbsp almond milk
- ½ tsp sea salt

Instructions:

1. In a saucepan over medium heat, heat the coconut oil. Don't let it get too hot or the flour will instantly burn.
2. Add the coconut flour and whisk to make a thick paste.
3. Slowly whisk in the vegetable broth. Bring to a boil and cook for 4 minutes, or until thickened.
4. Reduce the heat to low. Add the almond milk and salt. Continue cooking until the desired consistency.
5. Serve warm.
6. Nutrients per serving: Carbohydrates – 2.8 g Fiber – 0.8 g Fat – 2.5 g Protein – 1.8 g Calories – 35

Apple Butter

Prep time: 10 minutes

Cooking time: 3 hours **Servings:** 24

Ingredients:

- 4 pounds apples, peeled, chopped
- 2 cups fresh apple juice
- Tbsp lemon juice, freshly squeezed
- packets stevia
- 1 tsp cinnamon
- 1 vanilla bean, split lengthwise, deseeded
- Pinch ground cloves

Instructions:

1. Add the apples, apple juice, and lemon juice to a pot. Bring to a simmer and cook for 1 hour, until soft. Remove from the heat and cool slightly.
2. In a blender, purée the apples until smooth.
3. Take the puree out. Add the stevia, cinnamon, vanilla bean seeds, and cloves to the apples. Cook for an additional 2 hours, stirring frequently.
4. Cool the apple butter. Transfer to an airtight container and refrigerate.
5. Nutrients per serving: Carbohydrates – 12.9 g Fiber – 1.9 g Fat – 0.2 g Protein – 0.2 g Calories – 49

Sun-Dried Tomato Sauce

Prep time: 10 minutes

Cooking time: 0 minutes

Servings: 4

Ingredients:

- cup cherry tomatoes, halved
- ½ cup tightly packed sun-dried tomatoes
- Tbsp coconut oil
- ⅓ cup fresh basil
- 1 Tbsp tomato paste
- 1 tsp sea salt
- 1 tsp garlic powder

Instructions:

1. In a food processor, combine all Ingredients:.
2. Pulse to combine.
3. Nutrients per serving: Carbohydrates – 6.1 g Fiber – 1.5 g Fat – 12.2 g Protein – 1.4 g Calories – 132

Enchilada Sauce

Prep time: 5 minutes

Cooking time: 26 minutes

Servings: 8

Ingredients:

- 2 Tbsp coconut oil
- 2 Tbsp coconut flour
- 2 Tbsp chili powder
- 2 cups water
- 8-oz can tomato paste
- 1 tsp garlic powder
- ½ tsp cumin
- ½ tsp onion powder
- ½ tsp sea salt
- ¼ tsp red pepper flakes

Instructions:

1. In a pot over medium heat, heat the coconut oil, coconut flour, and chili powder. Cook for 1 minute.
2. Add the water, tomato paste, garlic powder, cumin, onion powder, salt, and red pepper flakes, to taste. Bring the mixture to a simmer and cook for 25 minutes, stirring occasionally.
3. Serve warm
4. Nutrients per serving: Carbohydrates – 8.3 g Fiber – 1.6 g Fat – 3.6 g Protein – 1.8 g Calories – 68

Alkaline Salsa Mexicana

The Salsa Mexicana is tasteful, delicious, healthy, and alkaline. It is highly nutritious, as some of the **Ingredients:** used in preparation are tomatoes, cilantro, lime juice, garlic, and chili.

Garlic is known to contain compounds that are highly medicinal in nature e.g., it contains compounds that help combat common cold, reduce blood pressure, improve cholesterol levels, and prevent dementia, etc.

Tomatoes are known to have anti-carcinogenic properties e.g., the chlorogenic acid and coumaric acid found in tomatoes are known to combat nitrosamines, the carcinogenic properties of cigarettes.

The Vitamin A found in tomatoes are also known to boost eye vision. Other health benefits of tomatoes include; it aids digestion, helps to lower hypertension, helps to maintain the skin, hair, teeth, and bones.

Cilantro, on the other hand, helps rid the body of metals, reduces anxiety, supports heart health, soothes skin irritation, prevents inflammation, and protects against urinary tract infections.

Enjoy this healthy recipe

Servings: one (1) bowl

Ingredients:

- Cayenne Pepper, one (1) pinch
- Spring onions, two (2)
- Tomatoes (big), three (3)
- Cilantro (a handful)
- Juice of lime, one (1)
- Organic or sea salt (one pinch)
- Chilies (green), two (2)
- Garlic, two (2) cloves

Directions:

1. Chop garlic cloves in tiny pieces, cut the chilies in small pieces, cut the onions in rings, and put the tomatoes in small cubes.
2. There are two ways you can about it, depend on how you prefer your salsa (either smooth or chunky).
3. For a smooth salsa; add all the Ingredients: in a mixing pan and mix well.
4. Empty the mix in a food processor and blast for a few seconds.
5. Add salt and pepper to taste.
6. Serve.
7. However, for a chunky salsa; add all Ingredients: together in a mixing bowl and mix properly.
8. Add salt and pepper to taste.
9. Serve.

Soy Cucumber Shake

The Soy cucumber shake is easy to make, simple and highly nutritious. The highly nutritious **Ingredients:** that make up this shake include vanilla, cucumber, coconut milk, and soy milk.

Vanilla is rich in antioxidants, meaning it contains healing properties right at the gene-level. It also contains properties that boost the immune system, prevent acne, cure respiratory conditions, and aid digestion.

Cucumbers are also known to contain antioxidants, aid weight loss, promote body hydration, and lower blood sugar.

Soy milk helps women in the sense that it helps relieve postmenopausal issues, provides relief from Osteoporosis, controls obesity, and lowers cholesterol.

This is a supremely rich, healthy and alkaline recipe.

Ingredients:

- Vanilla (organic), one (1) teaspoon
- Small cucumbers (shredded), two (2)
- Fresh coconut milk (unsweetened), 50ml
- Fresh soy milk (unsweetened), 500ml
- Ice Cubes made with alkaline water, six (6) – eight (8) cubes

Directions:

1. Add all the Ingredients: and blast for until it is smooth to consistency.
2. Serve.

Tofu Salad Dressing

Tofu salad dressing is easy to make, quick, healthy, and above all, alkaline.

Some of the **Ingredients:** used in this recipe include tofu, stevia powder, sea salt, and herbs. Tofu is known to contain properties that help maintain cardiovascular health, ease menopause symptoms in women, prevent osteoporosis, and boost brain health, to mention but a few

Stevia controls diabetes and weight loss, prevents certain types of cancer, lowers cholesterol levels, as well as promotes skin health.

Enjoy

Ingredients:

- Stevia powder, One (1) teaspoon
- Tofu, 100g
- Alkaline water, Five (5) tablespoons
- Random spices and herbs of your choice
- Sea salt, ½ teaspoon

Directions:

1. Add all Ingredients: in a food processor and process until it is fine to consistency.
2. Enjoy it with salad.

Millet Spread

Millet spread is easy to make, tasteful, quick and extremely healthy. The **Ingredients:** here include olive oil, millet, vegetable stock, and other herbs, vegetables and white onions.

Olive oil, as we know, contains large amounts of antioxidants and contains high anti-inflammatory properties. It possesses abilities that help prevent stroke, protect the health against diseases, and prevent against Diabetes type 2.

White onions are known to prevent blood clots, which in turn helps heart health. Quercetin, are known anti-carcinogenic agents present in white onion. The high amount of sulfur in white onion makes it highly anti-inflammatory. White onions generally regulate blood sugar, support digestive health, and improve bone density.

Enjoy this awesome recipe.

Ingredients:

- Pepper, one (1) pinch
- White onion (big), one (1)
- Millet, one (1) cup
- Any garden herb of your choice, one (1) teaspoon
- Virgin olive oil (cold pressed extra), one (1) tablespoon
- Alkaline water, two (2) cups
- Organic/sea salt, one (1) pinch
- Yeast free vegetable stock, one (1) teaspoon

Directions:

1. Get a small pot over medium heat, add water, the vegetable stock, and millet and boil for ten minutes, and put the pot aside for some minutes.
2. In a different pan, add oil and stir fry the roughly chopped onion.
3. Once that is done, add the stir-fried onion to the millet.
4. Mix properly, then add salt and pepper to taste.
5. Place it in a mixer and puree for 40 seconds.
6. Serve.

Alkaline Eggplant Dip

The beautiful thing about eggplants is that they are not only alkaline-rich, they are also antioxidant, nutritious, and tasty. Some of their health benefits include; they help to regulate blood pressure, as well as helping keep the body hydrated.

Generally, it is a known fact that garlic contains highly medicinal compounds that help the human body fight symptoms such as common cold and running nose. Other health benefits of garlic include the reduction of blood pressure and the prevention of dementia.

Parsley, on the other hand, contains compounds that help them beat inflammation, improve the immune system, and reduce cancer risk.

Ingredients:

- Garlic, two (2) cloves
- Lemon juice (fresh), five (5) tablespoons
- Parsley (a handful)
- Cayenne pepper (a pinch)
- Organic salt or sea salt (a pinch)
- Eggplant (700g)
- Sesame paste, six (6) tablespoons

Directions:

1. First of all, you should preheat the oven to around 400 degrees Fahrenheit.
2. Wash the eggplants and use a fork to prick several places.
3. Place in the oven on a grid and heat for between thirty to forty minutes.
4. While this is going one, chop the parsley and garlic and set aside.
5. Take off the eggplant from the oven after forty minutes and allow it to cool.
6. Once it's cooled, peel the eggplants and scoop out the pulp.
7. Chop the pulp finely on a chopping board and empty in a mixing bowl.
8. In the mixing bowl, sprinkle the lemon juice and mash with a spoon until it becomes smooth.
9. Finally, add garlic, the parsley, and the sesame paste.
10. Season with pepper and salt to taste.
11. Serve.

Coriander Spread

This easy to make, quick and healthy coriander spread is made with fresh coriander and other food items such as chili, ginger, lime juice, water, and salt. These **Ingredients:** are known to individually contain nutrients and minerals that are highly helpful for the continued well-being of the human body.

Coriander leaves have come a long way both as a food ingredient and as a nutritious element that provides numerous nutrients for the human body. For example, they are known to reduce skin inflammation, relieve skin disorders, lower cholesterol levels, and regulate blood pressure.

Other health benefits of coriander leaves include; prevention of menstrual disorders in women, protection against mouth ulcers, salmonella protection and treatment of diarrhea, etc.

Lime juice improves the taste of food, aids digestion, contains anti-carcinogenic properties, promotes weight loss, and improves the immune system. Other health benefits include; reduction of blood sugar, the prevention of kidney stones, and the reduction of heart disease.

Enjoy your alkaline coriander spread.

Ingredients:

- Chili (green), 1-2
- Ginger (fresh), ½ inch
- Lime juice (fresh), two (2) tablespoons
- Coconut flakes (freshly grated), one (1) cup
- Coriander leaves (fresh), three (3) cups
- Alkaline water, four (4) tablespoons
- Organic or sea salt, one pinch

Directions:

1. Chop the ginger, chili and coriander leaves.
2. Add all Ingredients: in a blender and blend until the mix is smooth to consistency.
3. When that is done, you can add some organic or sea salt and season to taste.
4. Lastly, it is recommended that you put the mix in the fridge for about an hour.
5. Serve.

Polo Salad Dressing

The Polo Salad dressing is a healthy recipe that is aimed at adding more taste and vigor to your dining table. It is easy to make, quick, and nutrient rich.

Dates, which is one of the **Ingredients:** in this meal does not only add sweetness to this recipe, it also contains far more health benefits including; the supply of fiber to the body, control of blood sugar and prevention of osteoporosis. Other effects are; it improves brain health, contains antioxidants, and helps women during childbirth.

Lemon juice is known for the distinct taste and flavor it brings to the table. Other than that, its health benefits are also well known, including; the supply of vitamin C, which helps reduce stroke and other cardiovascular diseases, improvement of skin quality, and body hydration.

Miso aids digestion, boosts the immune system, contains anti-inflammatory properties, and promotes heart health.

Ingredients:

- Dates, two (2)
- Juice of lemon, (½ lemon)
- Alkaline water, ½ cup
- Cayenne pepper and sea salt, one (1) dash
- Extra virgin oil (cold pressed), 1/3 cup
- Miso, one (1) tablespoon

Directions:

1. Add all Ingredients: in a blender and blast until the mix is smooth to consistency.
2. You can add more salt and pepper if desired.
3. Serve.

Citrus Alkaline Salad Dressing

The citrus salad dressing is highly alkaline, tasteful, easy to make, and nutrient rich. This recipe is a blend of lime or lemon, pepper, basil, olive oil, oregano, garlic, rosemary, and cumin. The best part is that it is raw!

Lemon juice doesn't only add a distinct after taste to this recipe; it also comes fully loaded with health-related benefits such as improving body hydration, improving skin quality, promoting digestion, prevention of kidney stones, as well as aiding fresh breath.

The idea of adding Cumin to this recipe is primarily due to its spicy nature, as well as its ability to combine well with pepper and salt. However, on the health side, Cumin is a significant source of Iron, phenols, flavonoids, terpenes, and alkaloids. Cumin also helps prevent Diabetes, promote weight loss, and prevent food-borne diseases.

Oregano is a staple herb for dishes in many countries due to its unique and robust flavor. They are highly nutritious and are known to help fight bacteria, reduce viral infections, decrease inflammation, and are anti-carcinogenic.

Ingredients:

- Garlic powder, one (1) teaspoon
- Rosemary (dried), ¼ teaspoon
- Cumin (ground), ½ teaspoon
- Oregano (ground), ½ teaspoon
- Basil (dried), one (1) teaspoon
- Olive oil (cold pressed), ¾ cup
- Cayenne pepper and sea salt, one (1) dash
- Fresh lime or lemon juice, 1/3 cup

Directions:

1. Add all the Ingredients: in a blender and blast until the mix is smooth to consistency.
2. You can season with pepper and salt if desired.
3. Serve.

Avocado Spinach Dip

The Avocado Spinach Dip is an extraordinarily healthy and raw recipe. The highlight of this particular recipe is that it is highly alkaline, simple to make and tasty.

When you add Dil, avocado, garlic, spinach, Tahini, chili, pepper, and salt together in the right doses, you are guaranteed to come up with something worthwhile and that is the case with the Avocado Spinach Dip.

As we know, Dil is medically known to prevent insomnia, promote digestion, maintain bone health, prevent excessive gas, as well as control diabetes. Other health effects of Dil are; it boosts immunity, calms hiccups, cures diarrhea, treats dysentery and relieves arthritis pain.

Avocado is rich in vitamins K, C, B5, B6, E, potassium, folate, and fiber. It helps lower cholesterol and triglyceride levels, helps to lower certain cancer risks, helps relieve arthritis symptoms, and supports weight loss.

Garlic combats the common cold, reduces blood pressure, controls cholesterol levels, and helps fight dementia.

Finally, Spinach improves eyesight, relieves symptoms of Hemophilia, controls blood pressure, strengthen s the muscles, and helps provide bone minerals. Other health benefits are; it aids the digestive system, prevents Atherosclerosis, and promotes fetal development.

Enjoy this tasty alkaline health recipe!

Ingredients:

- Dil, one (1) cup
- Avocado, one (1)
- Garlic, one (1) clove
- Parsley, one (1) cup
- Spinach (fresh), 150g
- Tahini, one (1) tablespoon
- Chili, one (1)
- Pepper and sea salt to taste

Directions:

1. Add all Ingredients: in a blender.
2. Blend until the mix turns creamy and smooth to consistency.
3. You can add pepper and salt to taste.
4. Serve.

Alkaline Vegetable Spread

The vegetable spread is healthy, alkaline, easy to make and quick. When you take a closer look at the **Ingredients:** that make up this recipe, you'll understand why it is on this list in the first place.

Let's look at the health benefits of each ingredient one after the other.

Pepper is typically used to improve the taste of food, but it also contains some compounds that are beneficial to the human body e.g., the capsaicin in peppers aid digestive tracts, pepper lowers cholesterol levels, relieves joint pain, improves metabolism and promotes weight loss, cures Psoriasis and fight fungal infections.

Tomatoes have anti-carcinogenic properties, promote skin health, and promote heart health.

Avocado helps reduce triglyceride and cholesterol levels, helps lower certain cancer risks, helps relieve arthritis symptoms, and supports weight loss.

Bean sprouts have compounds that reduce anxiety caused by excessive stress; they also help maintain good eyesight, boost the immune system, promote heart health, and build strong bones.

Celery helps lower inflammation, reduces high cholesterol, reduces high blood pressure, and prevents liver diseases, fight infections, and cures bloating. Other health benefits include; prevention of ulcers, reduction of urinary tract infections, and reduction of cancer risks.

Alfalfa sprouts help to heal open wounds, improve bone health, prevent iron deficiency, aid weight loss and help fight cold sores.

Sunflower seeds improve cholesterol levels, support bone health, control blood sugar, promote healthy detoxification and support skin health. It also helps good mood, aid weight loss, fights hypertension, and promote hair growth.

Cucumber promotes hydration, contains antioxidants, aid weight loss, and lowers blood sugar.

Enjoy this recipe.

Ingredients:

- Pepper, one (1) pinch
- Tomato, one (1)
- Avocado, one (1)
- Yeast free vegetable stock, one (1) teaspoon
- Bean sprouts, ½ cup
- Celery stalk, one (1)
- Alfalfa sprouts, ½ cup
- Sunflower seeds, one (1) handful
- Organic salt or sea salt, one (1) pinch
- Any garden herb of your choice, one (1) teaspoon
- Extra virgin oil (cold pressed), one (1) tablespoon
- Cucumber ½

Directions:

1. Depending on how you like your spread, you can either puree or not. Since we want this spread to be chunky, we won't puree.
2. So, chop the alfalfa sprouts, cucumber, tomato, celery, and bean sprout into tiny pieces.
3. Get a mixing bowl and toss all the chopped Ingredients: into it.
4. Add sunflower seeds and mix properly.
5. Mash the avocado and add in a separate bowl, along with the olive oil, vegetable stock, lemon juice, salt and pepper, and herbs.
6. Stir until it forms a creamy paste.
7. Finally, mix the mashed avocado cream with the vegetables.
8. Stir consistently until all Ingredients: are mixed properly.
9. Refrigerate for about an hour.
10. Serve.

Alkaline sunflower sauce

The Alkaline Sunflower Sauce is straightforward and easy to make, contains healthy food items, and tastes extremely good.

One important thing to always remember about alkaline foods is that they are specifically meant to add value to your health. So if a meal doesn't have nutrients that would alkalize your body pH and improve your health, then it is not an alkaline diet.

The **Ingredients:** that make up this recipe are natural, raw, and consist of numerous benefits to human health. For example, tomatoes have anti-carcinogenic properties; they also improve heart health and aid skin health.

Sunflower seeds control cholesterol levels, aid bone health, regulate blood sugar, support skin health, and aid detoxification.

Garlic helps reduce blood pressure, combat common cold, improves cholesterol levels and improves athletic performance, etc.

Olive oil contains significant amounts of anti-oxidants, it is highly anti-inflammatory, helps prevent strokes, promotes heart health, and reduces risks of diabetes type 2.

Pepper mitigates migraines, relieves joint pain, reduces certain cancer risks and improves metabolism.

Ingredients:

- Tomato, one (1)
- Sunflower seeds, 200g
- Red pepper, one (1)
- Garlic, one (1) clove
- Extra virgin olive oil (cold pressed), one (teaspoon)
- Pepper (a pinch)
- Organic salt or sea salt (a pinch)
- Any herb of your choice

Directions:

1. Note: Before you start this process, you should soak the sunflower seeds for about four (4) hours before commencement.
2. Add all Ingredients: in a blender and blast till the mix turns into a smooth cream.
3. Add your favorite herbs, pepper and salt to taste.
4. Serve.

Almond-Red Bell Pepper Dip

The Almond-Red Bell Pepper Dip is a decent and straightforward alkaline mix that is rich in natural nutrients and minerals. The Ingredients: can be sourced from your local stores and markets, so you should try it out sometimes.

It is very healthy! A look at the Ingredients: will give you a sneak peek of the benefits of the dip to human health.

Garlic is known to combat common cold, improve cholesterol levels, and reduce blood pressure.

Red pepper fights fungal infections, flu, and colds. It contains anti-carcinogenic properties, control migraines, cures Psoriasis and improves heart health.

Almonds are loaded with fiber, protein, vitamin E, manganese, magnesium, and phytic acid. They contain antioxidants, control blood sugar, lower cholesterol levels and mitigate blood pressure.

Ingredients:

- Garlic, 2-3 cloves
- Sea salt, one (1) pinch
- Cayenne pepper, one (1) pinch
- Extra virgin olive oil (cold pressed), one (1) tablespoon
- Almonds, 60g
- Red bell pepper, 280g

Directions:

1. First of all, cook garlic and pepper until they are soft.
2. Add all Ingredients: in a blender and blend until the mix becomes smooth and creamy.
3. Finally, add pepper and salt to taste.
4. Serve.

Conclusion

With the single aim of introducing readers to the alkaline diet and showing them how to implement it daily, the author of this cookbook shares a wide range of unique and flavorsome recipes along with a comprehensive alkaline diet guide. Give each section a thorough read and discover basic tips, suggestions, and techniques to incorporate more alkaline foods into your routine diet.